"Deliciously Healthy Meals: A Cookbook for Alzheimer's Care and Nutrition for Seniors"

Trina H. Nelson

Table of Contents

Introduction
    Overview of Alzheimer's disease and its impact on nutrition
    The importance of a healthy diet for seniors with Alzheimer's

Chapter 1: Healthy Eating for Seniors
    Introduction to Nutrition and Aging
    Role of Nutrition in Alzheimer's disease.
    Dietary Management Strategies
    Nutritional Recommendations for Alzhemier's Patients.
        Basic Nutritional Needs
        Disease-Specific Needs
    Nutritional Recommendations for Alzheimer's Patients
    Identifying and addressing malnutrition in seniors with Alzheimer's

Chapter 2: Meal Planning and Preparing for Alzheimer's Care
    Meal Planning Considerations for Alzheimer's Patients.
    Creating Nutrient-Rich Meals for Alzheimer's Patients.
    The benefits of meal planning for Alzheimer's care
    Adapting recipes for seniors with swallowing difficulties.
    Tips for making meals more visually appealing.
    Incorporating foods that may improve cognitive function.
    Tips for Incorporating Cognitive-Enhancing Foods Into an Alzheimer's Patient's Diet

Chapter 3: Deliciously Healthy Recipes for Seniors
    Breakfast Recipes
    Lunch Recipes.
    Dinner recipes.
    Snack and Dessert Recipes.

Chapter 4: Special Dietary Needs for Seniors
    Low-Sodium Recipes

Gluten-Free Recipes
Low-Fat Recipe
Sugar-Free Recipes
4-weeks Sample Meal Plan
    Week 1
    Week 2
    Week 3
    Week 4

Conclusion

Introduction

Welcome to "Deliciously Mindful: A Cookbook for Alzheimer's Caregivers and Seniors." This cookbook is designed specifically for caregivers and families of seniors who have been diagnosed with Alzheimer's disease. As you may already know, Alzheimer's is a progressive brain disorder that affects memory, thinking, and behavior. It is the most common cause of dementia among older adults and it affects millions of people worldwide.

Caring for a loved one with Alzheimer's is a challenging and often overwhelming task. One of the most important aspects of care is ensuring that they receive proper nutrition. As the disease progresses, seniors with Alzheimer's may have difficulty swallowing, lose their sense of taste or appetite, or become confused about what to eat. As a result, they may not get the nutrients they need to maintain their health. This can lead to malnutrition and other health problems.

That's where this cookbook comes in. We have compiled a collection of delicious and nutritious recipes that are easy to prepare and cater to the specific needs of seniors with Alzheimer's. We understand that mealtime can be stressful for caregivers and families, so we've included tips and suggestions on how to make mealtime more enjoyable and less stressful for both the caregiver and the senior with Alzheimer's.

In addition to providing recipes, this cookbook also includes information on the role of nutrition in Alzheimer's disease and nutritional recommendations for Alzheimer's patients. We also discuss ways to identify and address malnutrition in seniors with Alzheimer's.

This cookbook is not just a collection of recipes, but it's a guide for caregivers and families to understand the importance of nutrition in Alzheimer's care and how to provide nutritious meals for their loved ones with the disease. The recipes included in this cookbook are easy to prepare, delicious and most importantly tailored to the needs of Alzheimer's patients.

We hope this cookbook will be a valuable resource for you and your loved one. We understand that caring for a loved one with Alzheimer's is a difficult journey, but we believe that small things like enjoying a delicious and nutritious meal together can make a big difference in the overall well-being of both the caregiver and the senior with Alzheimer's. So, let's dive into the world of nutritious and delicious meals.

We hope that this cookbook will not only help you provide nutritious meals for your loved one with Alzheimer's but also bring some joy and comfort to your meal times together.

Overview of Alzheimer's disease and its impact on nutrition

Alzheimer's disease is a degenerative brain ailment that impairs memory, thinking, and behavior.. It is the most common cause of dementia among older adults and it affects millions of people worldwide.

The exact causes of Alzheimer's disease are not yet fully understood, but it is believed to be a combination of genetic, environmental, and lifestyle factors. The disease typically develops in people over the age of 65, but early-onset Alzheimer's can occur in people as young as their 30s or 40s.

As the disease progresses, individuals with Alzheimer's may have difficulty with daily activities such as dressing, bathing, and eating. They may also experience memory loss, disorientation, and changes in mood and behavior.

One of the most significant impacts of Alzheimer's disease on nutrition is that it can affect a person's ability to eat and enjoy food. As the disease progresses, individuals with Alzheimer's may lose their sense of taste or appetite, or become confused about what to eat. They may also have difficulty swallowing, which can lead to malnutrition and other health problems.

Malnutrition can occur when a person with Alzheimer's is not getting the right balance of nutrients, or not getting enough calories. This can lead to weight loss, weakness, and an increased risk of infections and other health problems. Malnutrition can also make the symptoms of Alzheimer's worse, by making it harder for a person to think and communicate.

Additionally, some medications used to treat Alzheimer's can also affect a person's appetite, making it difficult for them to eat and get the nutrients they need.

To address these issues, it's important for caregivers and families of individuals with Alzheimer's to understand the importance of nutrition in Alzheimer's care and to provide nutritious meals that are easy to eat and enjoy. This can include adapting recipes to make them more visually appealing, incorporating foods that may improve cognitive function, and providing foods in a texture that is easy to swallow.

It's also important for caregivers and families to monitor for signs of malnutrition in their loved ones with Alzheimer's, and to work with a healthcare professional if they suspect that their loved one is not getting the nutrition they need.

In conclusion, Alzheimer's disease can have a significant impact on nutrition and can affect a person's ability to eat and enjoy food. Caregivers and families of individuals with Alzheimer's should be aware of the importance of nutrition in Alzheimer's care and should work to provide nutritious meals that are easy to eat and enjoy. They should also monitor for signs of malnutrition in their loved one and work with a healthcare professional if they suspect malnutrition.

The importance of a healthy diet for seniors with Alzheimer's

A healthy diet is essential for seniors with Alzheimer's disease, as it can help to improve their overall health and well-being. As the disease progresses, individuals with Alzheimer's may have difficulty with daily activities such as dressing, bathing, and eating. They may also experience memory loss, disorientation, and changes in mood and behavior. These symptoms can make it difficult for seniors with Alzheimer's to maintain a healthy diet, but it is important for caregivers and families to understand the importance of nutrition in Alzheimer's care and to work to provide nutritious meals that are easy to eat and enjoy.

One of the most significant impacts of Alzheimer's disease on nutrition is that it can affect a person's ability to eat and enjoy food. As the disease progresses, individuals with Alzheimer's may lose their sense of taste or appetite, or become confused about what to eat. They may also have difficulty swallowing, which can lead to malnutrition and other health problems. Malnutrition can occur when a person with Alzheimer's is not getting the right balance of nutrients, or not getting enough calories. This can lead to weight loss, weakness, and an increased risk of infections and other health problems. Malnutrition can also make the symptoms of Alzheimer's worse, by making it harder for a person to think and communicate.

In addition to the physical effects of malnutrition, seniors with Alzheimer's may also experience emotional and social effects. They may feel isolated and depressed, and may have difficulty enjoying their food or participating in social events. Caregivers and families can help to address these issues by providing nutritious meals that are easy to eat and enjoy, and by making mealtime a social and enjoyable experience.

To ensure that seniors with Alzheimer's receive the nutrition they need, it is important for caregivers and families to understand the nutritional needs of individuals with Alzheimer's and to work with a healthcare professional to create a personalized meal plan. A healthy diet for seniors with Alzheimer's should include a balance of carbohydrates, proteins, and healthy fats. It should also include a variety of fruits and vegetables, as well as adequate hydration.

Carbohydrates provide energy and are an important source of calories for seniors with Alzheimer's. Whole grains, such as whole wheat bread and brown rice, are a good source of carbohydrates and provide important nutrients such as fiber, vitamins, and minerals. Proteins are also essential for maintaining muscle mass and strength, and can be found in lean meats, fish, and plant-based proteins such as beans and lentils. Healthy fats, such as those found in nuts, seeds, and avocados, can also be beneficial for seniors with Alzheimer's, as they can help to improve cognitive function and support healthy brain function.

Fruits and vegetables are also an important part of a healthy diet for seniors with Alzheimer's. They are rich in vitamins, minerals, and antioxidants, which can help to protect against disease and promote overall health. In addition to providing important nutrients, fruits and vegetables can also provide a variety of textures and flavors, which can be beneficial for seniors with Alzheimer's who may have difficulty with taste or appetite.

Adequate hydration is also important for seniors with Alzheimer's. As the disease progresses, individuals with Alzheimer's may have difficulty remembering to drink enough fluids, which can lead to dehydration. Caregivers and families can help to ensure that their loved one with Alzheimer's stays hydrated by providing fluids throughout the day and by encouraging them to drink fluids with meals.

It's also important to keep in mind that some medications used to treat Alzheimer's can also affect a person's appetite, making it difficult for them to eat and get the nutrients they need. Caregivers and families should work with their loved one's healthcare provider to ensure that their medications do not interfere with their ability to eat and receive proper nutrition. They should also monitor for any side effects of medications that may affect appetite or digestion and report them to the healthcare provider.

Another important aspect of nutrition for seniors with Alzheimer's is the texture of food. As the disease progresses, some seniors may develop swallowing difficulties, known as dysphagia, which can make it difficult for them to eat solid foods. Caregivers and families can work with a healthcare professional to create a meal plan that includes soft, easy-to-swallow foods, such as pureed fruits and vegetables, soups, and stews.

Creating a personalized meal plan for a senior with Alzheimer's can be challenging, but it is important for the overall health and well-being of the senior. Caregivers and families should work with a healthcare professional, such as a registered dietitian, to create a meal plan that meets the specific needs of their loved one. This can include taking into account any dietary restrictions or allergies, as well as any physical or cognitive limitations.

In conclusion, a healthy diet is essential for seniors with Alzheimer's disease. As the disease progresses, individuals with Alzheimer's may have difficulty with daily activities such as dressing, bathing, and eating. They may also experience memory loss, disorientation, and changes in mood and behavior. These symptoms can make it difficult for seniors with Alzheimer's to maintain a healthy diet, but it is important for caregivers and families to understand the importance of nutrition in Alzheimer's care and to work to provide nutritious meals that are easy to eat and enjoy. Caregivers and families should also monitor for signs of malnutrition in their loved one and work with a healthcare professional if they suspect malnutrition.

Chapter 1: Healthy Eating for Seniors

Eating a healthy diet can be an important part of maintaining a healthy lifestyle for seniors, particularly those with Alzheimer's disease. Eating nutritious foods can help seniors stay strong and mentally alert, helping to slow down the progression of the disease.

The best diet for seniors with Alzheimer's is one that is rich in fruits and vegetables, whole grains, lean proteins, and healthy fats. Fruits and vegetables are packed with antioxidants and other vitamins and minerals that can help protect the brain from damage and inflammation caused by the disease. Whole grains provide fiber and B vitamins that are important for maintaining cognitive function. Lean proteins such as beans, fish, and poultry provide essential amino acids and are important for preventing muscle loss. Healthy fats from fish, nuts, and seeds provide essential fatty acids that are important for brain health.

It is also important for seniors to stay hydrated by drinking plenty of water throughout the day. Dehydration can lead to confusion and cognitive decline, and can worsen the symptoms of Alzheimer's.

It is best to avoid processed, sugary, and salty foods, as these can lead to weight gain and an increased risk of developing diabetes and other chronic diseases. It is also important to limit caffeine and alcohol consumption, as these can interfere with sleep and further disrupt cognitive function.

By making healthy eating choices and maintaining an active lifestyle, seniors with Alzheimer's can help slow down the progression of the disease and enjoy a higher quality of life.

Introduction to Nutrition and Aging

Nutrition and aging are important topics when considering Alzheimer's disease, a neurological disorder that affects memory, thinking, and behavior. As people age, their bodies become less efficient and more susceptible to age-related diseases such as Alzheimer's. Nutrition plays a major role in how the body ages, and how well it can protect itself against age-related diseases. Nutrition can provide the body with the necessary nutrients to help maintain cognitive and physical health, which can reduce the risk of developing Alzheimer's disease.

Nutrition is important for aging because it provides the body with the necessary nutrients to maintain health and protect against age-related diseases. Research has shown that a healthy diet that includes plenty of fruits and vegetables, whole grains, healthy fats, and lean proteins can help reduce the risk of developing Alzheimer's disease. Eating a variety of foods, including foods that contain antioxidants, can help protect the body from free radicals, which are molecules that can damage cells. Additionally, some studies have found that certain types of fats, such as Omega-3 fatty acids, can help protect the brain from age-related decline.

Nutrition is also important for aging because it can help keep the body strong and healthy. Eating a balanced diet that includes plenty of fruits and vegetables, whole grains, and lean proteins can help maintain muscle mass, which is important for keeping the body strong and agile as people age. Additionally, it is important to stay hydrated by drinking plenty of water, as dehydration can lead to fatigue and cognitive decline.

Overall, nutrition and aging are important topics when considering Alzheimer's disease. Eating a balanced diet and staying hydrated can help reduce the risk of developing the disease, and can also help maintain the body's strength and agility as people age. Taking steps to maintain good nutrition can help protect against age-related diseases, and can help keep the body functioning at its best.

Role of Nutrition in Alzheimer's disease.

The role of nutrition in Alzheimer's disease is complex and not yet fully understood. It is known, however, that proper nutrition is key in maintaining cognitive function and overall health. It is believed that nutrition may influence the progression of the disease in several ways. First, it may affect the physical structure of the brain. Research has shown that the brain needs certain nutrients, such as omega-3 fatty acids, to build and repair neural pathways. Omega-3 fatty acids are found in fish, nuts, and some vegetable oils. A diet low in these types of fatty acids has been linked to an increased risk of developing Alzheimer's disease.

In addition, nutrition may affect the progression of the disease by influencing inflammation in the brain. Inflammation is a natural part of the body's response to injury or infection, but chronic inflammation can have a damaging effect on the brain. Poor nutrition can lead to chronic inflammation, which has been linked to the development and progression of Alzheimer's disease.

Finally, nutrition may influence the progression of the disease by affecting the production of neurotransmitters. Neurotransmitters are chemicals in the brain that carry signals between neurons. Diet can influence the production of certain neurotransmitters, such as acetylcholine, which is involved in memory and learning. A diet low in certain nutrients, such as vitamin B12, can lead to a deficiency in neurotransmitters, which can contribute to the development and progression of Alzheimer's disease.

Dietary Management Strategies

There is no "cure" for Alzheimer's disease, but there are dietary management strategies that may help to slow its progression. The most important strategy is to ensure that the person with Alzheimer's disease is receiving all the nutrients they need to maintain their health. This means a balanced diet that includes a variety of fruits, vegetables, whole grains, lean proteins, and healthy fats.

It is also important to limit processed and refined foods, as well as foods high in added sugars and saturated fats. These foods can contribute to inflammation and the development of other chronic diseases, which can further contribute to the progression of Alzheimer's disease.

In addition to a balanced diet, supplementation may be beneficial. Certain nutrients, such as omega-3 fatty acids and vitamin B12, have been linked to a decreased risk of developing Alzheimer's disease. It is important to talk to a doctor before starting any supplement regimen, as some supplements may interact with medications or have other adverse effects.

Nutritional Recommendations for Alzhemier's Patients.

The nutritional needs of Alzheimer's patients can be divided into two categories: basic nutritional needs and disease-specific needs.

Basic Nutritional Needs

First, Alzheimer's patients have the same basic nutritional needs as any other person. These include the consumption of a balanced diet with adequate amounts of carbohydrates, proteins, fats, vitamins, and minerals. This type of diet should include a variety of fruits, vegetables, lean proteins, whole grains, healthy fats, and dairy. Additionally, it should be low in sugar, salt, and saturated fat.

Disease-Specific Needs

Second, Alzheimer's patients have specific dietary needs related to the disease itself. These needs are as follows:

- High intake of antioxidant-rich foods: Antioxidants help protect the brain from damage caused by free radicals. Foods that are high in antioxidants include dark leafy greens, berries, nuts, and spices such as turmeric.

- Low intake of processed and refined foods: Processed and refined foods are high in added sugars and unhealthy fats, which can worsen cognitive decline.

- High intake of omega-3 fatty acids: Omega-3 fatty acids help to reduce inflammation, which is associated with cognitive decline. Foods that are high in omega-3s include fatty fish, walnuts, and flaxseed.

- Low intake of sodium: High sodium intake can lead to inflammation and dehydration, both of which can worsen cognitive decline.

Nutritional Recommendations for Alzheimer's Patients

Based on the nutritional needs of Alzheimer's patients, the following recommendations can be made to help them maintain their health and manage the progression of their condition:

- Eat a balanced diet: Eating a balanced diet with adequate amounts of carbohydrates, proteins, fats, vitamins, and minerals is important for maintaining overall health.

- Eat plenty of fruits and vegetables: Fruits and vegetables are high in antioxidants and other essential nutrients that can help protect the brain from damage.

- Limit processed and refined foods: Processed and refined foods are high in added sugars and unhealthy fats, which can worsen cognitive decline.

- Eat foods high in omega-3 fatty acids: Omega-3 fatty acids help to reduce inflammation, which is associated with cognitive decline.

- Limit sodium intake: High sodium intake can lead to inflammation and dehydration, both of which can worsen cognitive decline.

- Stay hydrated: Staying hydrated is important for overall health, as well as for avoiding dehydration and inflammation.

Identifying and addressing malnutrition in seniors with Alzheimer's

Malnutrition is a serious issue that is especially prevalent among seniors with Alzheimer's. While it is a common problem, it is often overlooked by caregivers and medical professionals. The good news is that it is possible to identify and address malnutrition in seniors with Alzheimer's. With the right interventions, seniors with Alzheimer's can stay healthy and maintain their nutritional status.

Malnutrition in seniors with Alzheimer's can be caused by a variety of factors, including a lack of appetite, difficulty eating due to physical challenges, difficulty swallowing, inability to recognize hunger, and even a lack of access to healthy food. Malnutrition can lead to a variety of health complications, including increased risk of infection, poor wound healing, increased risk of falls, and even death. It is important to recognize the signs of malnutrition in order to intervene and address the problem.

Common signs of malnutrition in seniors with Alzheimer's include extreme weight loss, changes in appetite, and changes in energy levels. If a senior with Alzheimer's is exhibiting any of these signs, it is important to speak to their doctor right away. The doctor can evaluate them and determine if they need to be referred to a nutritionist. A nutritionist can evaluate the senior's nutritional status and create a personalized nutrition plan that meets their needs.

In addition to medical intervention, there are several ways that caregivers can help address malnutrition in seniors with Alzheimer's. One of the most important steps is to ensure that the senior has access to healthy, nutritious food. This can be accomplished by providing meals that are high in protein, fiber, and other essential nutrients. It is also important to ensure that the senior is eating regularly, as this can help maintain a healthy weight.

Caregivers can also help seniors with Alzheimer's by providing them with food that is easy to eat and digest. This can include soft foods, finger foods, and pureed foods. Caregivers can also make mealtime a pleasant experience, as seniors with Alzheimer's may forget to eat or may not want to eat if mealtime is not enjoyable. It is also important to provide a variety of foods to ensure that the senior is getting all the necessary nutrients.

Finally, caregivers should also ensure that the senior is staying hydrated. Dehydration can further exacerbate malnutrition in seniors with Alzheimer's, so it is important to make sure they are drinking plenty of fluids. Caregivers should also be aware that certain medications can cause dehydration, so it is important to speak to the doctor or pharmacist about any potential side effects.

Malnutrition in seniors with Alzheimer's is a serious issue, but it is one that can be addressed with the right interventions. With the help of medical professionals and caregivers, seniors with Alzheimer's can receive the nutrition they need to stay healthy.

Chapter 2: Meal Planning and Preparing for Alzheimer's Care

Meal planning and preparation for those with Alzheimer's care is an important part of the caregiving process. Meal planning and preparation can help ensure that individuals with Alzheimer's get the nutrition they need, while also providing an enjoyable and meaningful activity for both the caregiver and the individual with Alzheimer's.

The first step in meal planning and preparation for those with Alzheimer's care is to assess the individual's food preferences and dietary needs. This may include consulting with a registered dietitian to make sure the individual is getting the right nutrients, as well as considering any special dietary requirements, such as low-sodium or low-fat diets. It is also important to consider the individual's food likes and dislikes.

Once the individual's nutritional needs and food preferences are determined, the caregiver can begin planning meals. It is important to plan meals that are nutritionally balanced and easy to prepare. For individuals with Alzheimer's, it is often helpful to plan meals around familiar foods and meals. This may include foods that the individual has enjoyed in the past, or that are traditional for the family or culture.

When preparing meals for individuals with Alzheimer's, it is important to keep the individual's abilities in mind. For those who are no longer able to feed themselves, caregivers should make sure that meals are cut into smaller pieces, and served in dishes that are easy to hold and manipulate. For those who are more independent, it is important to make sure that meals are presented in an attractive manner, and that food is served at the appropriate temperature.

Caregivers should also consider the individual's overall needs when planning meals. For example, those with Alzheimer's may have difficulty chewing or swallowing, so it is important to plan meals that are soft and easy to swallow. In addition, those with dementia may experience changes in appetite, so it is important to offer snacks throughout the day to ensure the individual is getting enough nutrition.

Finally, caregivers should provide a pleasant and calming environment for meals. It is important to allow plenty of time for the individual to eat, and to provide distractions and activities during meals, such as music or conversation. This can help create a pleasant and enjoyable atmosphere that can help individuals with Alzheimer's better enjoy their meals.

Meal planning and preparation for those with Alzheimer's care can be a challenging task, but it is an important part of providing quality care. With thoughtful planning and preparation, caregivers can ensure that individuals with Alzheimer's receive the nutrition they need, while also providing a meaningful and enjoyable activity.

Meal Planning Considerations for Alzheimer's Patients.

Meal planning for Alzheimer's patients can be a challenging task. As the disease progresses, it can be difficult for them to remember to eat healthy, or even to eat at all. Meal planning is important to ensure that they are getting the nutrition they need, and to help reduce the risk of malnutrition. Here are some considerations to keep in mind when meal planning for Alzheimer's patients.

1. Provide structure: Structure and routine are important for Alzheimer's patients, as it helps to reduce confusion and anxiety. Having a set schedule for meals can help provide a sense of stability and control.

2. Make the meal enjoyable: Mealtime should be a positive experience for Alzheimer's patients. Try to make the meal enjoyable by using colorful dishes and attractive presentation. Serve familiar foods that the patient enjoys, and consider trying new, interesting dishes as well.

3. Cater to their needs: Make sure to prepare meals that are tailored to the individual's needs. If they have difficulty swallowing, try to use softer foods or purees. If they are having difficulty with their appetite, experiment with different seasoning and flavors to make food more palatable.

4. Keep meals simple: Meals should be as simple as possible. Try to use few ingredients and limit choices to two or three options. Stick to familiar dishes and avoid complicated recipes.

5. Increase portion sizes: As Alzheimer's progresses, it can be difficult for patients to remember to eat. To compensate for this, increase portion sizes and serve meals regularly.

6. Provide assistance: Alzheimer's patients may need help with meal planning and preparation. Provide assistance with grocery shopping, menu planning, and cooking.

7. Serve balanced meals: Make sure to include all of the food groups in each meal. Aim for a balanced plate with a variety of fruits, vegetables, grains, proteins, and dairy products.

8. Consider dietary restrictions: If the patient has special dietary needs, cater the meals to their restrictions. Keep in mind any food allergies, sensitivities, or intolerances.

9. Include snacks: If the patient is having difficulty eating meals, include snacks throughout the day. Try offering healthy, nutrient-dense snacks such as nuts, yogurt, fruit, or cheese.

10. Monitor their weight: Monitor the patient's weight regularly to make sure they are getting the nutrition they need. If they are losing weight, increase portion sizes or offer more snacks.

Meal planning for Alzheimer's patients can be a difficult task, but with the right considerations, it can help ensure that they are getting the nutrition they need. Keep these tips in mind when meal planning for an Alzheimer's patient, and remember to make meals enjoyable and tailored to the individual's needs.

Creating Nutrient-Rich Meals for Alzheimer's Patients.

For those suffering from this condition, mealtime can be a difficult experience. As a caregiver, it is important to provide Alzheimer's patients with nutritious meals that will help them maintain their health and strength. Here are some tips for creating nutrient-rich meals for Alzheimer's patients.

The first step to creating nutrient-rich meals for Alzheimer's patients is to understand their nutritional needs. Alzheimer's patients require a balanced diet that includes plenty of fruits, vegetables, whole grains, lean proteins, and healthy fats. It is also important to provide adequate amounts of vitamins, minerals, and other essential nutrients. In addition, Alzheimer's patients may need to pay special attention to their sodium and cholesterol intake. It is important to speak to a physician or nutritionist to determine the exact nutritional requirements for an individual patient.

Once you have determined the nutritional needs of the patient, it is time to start planning meals. It is important to create meals that are both nutritious and appealing. Consider the patient's food preferences and create dishes that include their favorite foods. It is also important to incorporate foods that are high in antioxidants and other beneficial nutrients. These include leafy green vegetables, whole grains, nuts, and seeds.

When preparing meals for Alzheimer's patients, it is important to keep in mind that they may have difficulty with chewing and swallowing. To make meals easier to eat, it is best to serve foods that are soft and easy to chew. Soups, stews, and pureed foods are all great options. Another helpful tip is to use smaller plates and bowls. This will make it easier for the patient to manage their portions.

When creating nutritious meals for Alzheimer's patients, it is important to pay attention to portion sizes. Many Alzheimer's patients may not be able to recognize when they are full and may continue eating past the point of feeling full. To avoid this, serve smaller portions and allow the patient to ask for seconds if they are still hungry.

Finally, it is important to create a pleasant dining experience. Try to make mealtime a positive experience by incorporating pleasant conversations, music, or other activities. This can help make mealtime a more enjoyable experience for the patient.

Creating nutrient-rich meals for Alzheimer's patients can be a difficult task. However, with the right planning and preparation, it is possible to provide nutritious meals that are both healthy and enjoyable. By understanding the patient's nutritional needs, creating meals with appealing and easy-to-eat foods, and providing an enjoyable dining experience, caregivers can ensure that their patients are getting the nutrition they need.

The benefits of meal planning for Alzheimer's care

Meal planning is an important part of Alzheimer's care. It can help ensure that the person with Alzheimer's receives a balanced diet and enough calories and nutrients to remain healthy. Meal planning can also help make meals easier to prepare and may even provide a sense of structure and routine to the day.

Benefits of Meal Planning

1. Balanced Diet: Meal planning helps to ensure that the person with Alzheimer's receives the right amount of nutrients and calories for their age and activity level. Planning meals ahead of time can help to make sure that all of the food groups are included in the diet, such as dairy, proteins, fruits, veggies, and grains.

2. Easier Meal Preparation: Meal planning can help make meal preparation easier. When meals are planned ahead of time, it is easier to know exactly what ingredients to buy and how to prepare them. This can save time and energy in the kitchen.

3. Improved Nutrition: Meal planning can help to ensure that the person with Alzheimer's is receiving the right amount of nutrients to maintain their health. This can help to reduce the risk of malnutrition and other health complications associated with Alzheimer's.

4. Socialization: Meal planning can also help to create a sense of structure and routine for the day. This can provide a sense of comfort and familiarity, which can help to promote socialization and create an enjoyable mealtime experience.

5. Cost Savings: Meal planning can also help to save money. By planning meals ahead of time and sticking to a grocery list, it is easier to avoid overspending and waste.

6. Stress Reduction: Meal planning can help to reduce stress by taking away the need to quickly come up with meals and grocery lists each day. When meals are planned ahead of time, it is easier to just follow the plan and not have to worry about coming up with meals on the spot.

7. Improved Appetite: Meal planning can also help to stimulate the appetite. When meals are planned ahead of time, it is easier to plan meals that are both nutritious and enjoyable. This can help to encourage the person with Alzheimer's to eat more, which is important for maintaining their health.

8. Healthy Eating Habits: Meal planning can also help to instill healthy eating habits. By planning meals ahead of time, it is easier to control portion sizes and limit unhealthy snacks. This can help to promote healthier eating habits.

9. Variety: Meal planning can also help to ensure that the person with Alzheimer's is getting a variety of different foods. This can help to reduce boredom and ensure that they are getting all of the necessary vitamins and minerals.

10. Time Management: Meal planning can also help to save time. By planning meals ahead of time, it is easier to shop for the ingredients and prepare meals in a timely manner. This can help to make meal times easier and more efficient.

Adapting recipes for seniors with swallowing difficulties.

Adapting recipes for seniors with swallowing difficulties can be a challenge. It can be hard to know where to start, and how to make sure that the food is both nutritious and enjoyable. However, with a little bit of thought and creativity, it is possible to make meals that are both enjoyable and easy to swallow.

The first step to adapting recipes for seniors with swallowing difficulties is to choose the right ingredients. Soft or pureed foods are often the easiest to swallow, so it is important to select ingredients that are soft and easy to chew. This can include cooked fruits and vegetables, as well as softer proteins like fish, chicken, or eggs. Avoid crunchy or stringy ingredients, as these can be difficult to swallow.

It is also important to consider texture when adapting recipes for seniors with swallowing difficulties. Smooth textures are generally easier to swallow, so it is best to avoid chunky ingredients and sauces. Instead, focus on dishes that have a creamy, velvety texture. Soups, pureed vegetables, and mashed potatoes are all good options.

When adapting recipes for seniors with swallowing difficulties, it is important to consider flavor as well. Bland flavors can be difficult to swallow, so it is important to season dishes appropriately with herbs and spices. Marinating proteins in flavorful sauces can also help to make them easier to swallow. Aromatic herbs like rosemary, oregano, and thyme can be added to dishes to make them more flavorful.

When adapting recipes for seniors with swallowing difficulties, it is also important to consider portion size. Smaller portions are easier to swallow and easier to digest. It is best to divide recipes into multiple servings and serve them in individual portions. This will help to ensure that the food is not overwhelming and that the senior can easily swallow it.

Finally, it is important to make sure that the food is served warm. Cold foods can be difficult to swallow and can cause discomfort. When adapting recipes for seniors with swallowing difficulties, it is best to serve warm dishes that are at least room temperature.

Adapting recipes for seniors with swallowing difficulties can be challenging, but with a bit of thought and creativity, it is possible to create nutritious and enjoyable meals. By choosing soft ingredients, considering texture and flavor, and serving small portions, it is possible to make meals that are easy to swallow and enjoyable for seniors with swallowing difficulties.

Tips for making meals more visually appealing.

Making meals more visually appealing for Alzheimer's patients is an important part of providing them with the best care possible. Meals that are visually appealing can help stimulate the senses and promote positive dining experiences. This is particularly important for those with Alzheimer's disease, who often have difficulty recognizing tastes and textures. This guide will provide tips for making meals more visually appealing for Alzheimer's patients.

Here are some tips for Making Meals More Visually Appealing:

1. Use bright, contrasting colors. Incorporating bright and contrasting colors into meals can help make them more visually appealing. For example, adding red peppers and green leafy vegetables to a dish can make the meal more attractive.

2. Present the food in an interesting way. Presenting food in an interesting way can make it more visually appealing. For example, arranging food on a plate in a creative manner can make the meal more visually appealing.

3. Incorporate shapes and textures. Incorporating shapes and textures into meals can make them more visually appealing. For example,

adding vegetables cut into various shapes or adding crunchy items such as nuts or cereals can make the meal more attractive.

4. Use garnishes and decorations. Adding garnishes and decorations to meals can make them more visually appealing. For example, adding a sprig of parsley or a slice of lemon can make the meal look more attractive.

5. Use attractive dishes and utensils. Using attractive dishes and utensils can make meals more visually appealing. For example, using colorful plates or interesting utensils can make meals look more inviting.

6. Use aromatic ingredients. Incorporating aromatic ingredients into meals can make them more visually appealing. For example, adding herbs and spices to meals can make them more attractive.

7. Use seasonal fruits and vegetables. Incorporating seasonal fruits and vegetables into meals can make them more visually appealing. For example, using strawberries in the summer or squash in the winter can make meals look more attractive.

8. Present the food in a variety of ways. Presenting the food in a variety of ways can make meals more visually appealing. For

example, using different plating techniques can make meals look more interesting.

9. Use creative plate presentations. Using creative plate presentations can make meals more visually appealing. For example, arranging food in a circle or making a design with the food can make the meal look more attractive.

Making meals more visually appealing for Alzheimer's patients can help stimulate the senses and promote positive dining experiences. The tips in this guide can help make meals more visually appealing for Alzheimer's patients by incorporating bright and contrasting colors, presenting the food in an interesting way, incorporating shapes and textures, and using garnishes and decorations. Additionally, using attractive dishes and utensils, incorporating aromatic ingredients, using seasonal fruits and vegetables, presenting the food in a variety of ways, and using creative plate presentations can all help make meals more visually appealing.

Incorporating foods that may improve cognitive function.

The following types of foods may help improve cognitive function in Alzheimer's patients:

1. Omega-3 fatty acids: Omega-3 fatty acids, such as those found in fatty fish and some plant-based sources, are essential for proper brain health and may help reduce inflammation in the brain. Studies have shown that diets high in omega-3 fatty acids may help improve cognitive performance in Alzheimer's patients.

2. Antioxidant-rich foods: Antioxidants are compounds that help protect the body from free radical damage that can lead to cell damage. Foods that are rich in antioxidants, such as fruits and vegetables, may help reduce oxidative stress in the brain and improve cognitive performance in Alzheimer's patients.

3. Vitamin B12-rich foods: Vitamin B12 is an essential vitamin that helps the body produce red blood cells and is important for proper brain function. Vitamin B12 can be found in animal products, such as eggs, dairy, and meat, as well as some fortified foods. Studies have shown that diets high in vitamin B12 may help improve cognitive performance in Alzheimer's patients.

4. Curcumin: Curcumin is an active compound found in turmeric, a spice commonly used in Indian cooking. Studies have shown that curcumin may help reduce inflammation in the brain and improve cognitive performance in Alzheimer's patients.

5. Foods rich in Vitamin E: Vitamin E is an antioxidant that helps protect the body from free radical damage. Foods that are rich in

vitamin E, such as nuts, seeds, and vegetable oils, may help reduce oxidative stress in the brain and improve cognitive performance in Alzheimer's patients.

Tips for Incorporating Cognitive-Enhancing Foods Into an Alzheimer's Patient's Diet

1. Make meals colorful: Incorporating a variety of brightly colored fruits and vegetables into the diet of an Alzheimer's patient can provide a wealth of beneficial vitamins and minerals.

2. Focus on whole foods: Eating whole foods, such as lean proteins, fresh fruits and vegetables, healthy fats, and whole grains, can provide a variety of nutrients that may help improve cognitive function in Alzheimer's patients.

3. Spice it up: Adding spices and herbs to meals can add flavor and nutrients to the diet of an Alzheimer's patient. Spices, such as turmeric and ginger, may help reduce inflammation in the brain and improve cognitive performance.

4. Limit processed foods: Processed foods are generally high in sugar, salt, and unhealthy fats, and can contribute to inflammation in the brain. Limiting processed foods in the diet of an Alzheimer's patient can help improve cognitive performance.

5. Stay hydrated: Staying hydrated by drinking plenty of water throughout the day can help improve cognitive performance in Alzheimer's patients.

Chapter 3: Deliciously Healthy Recipes for Seniors

This chapter offers delicious and nutritious recipes designed to meet the needs of seniors with Alzheimer's disease. These recipes are easy to prepare and provide essential nutrients, such as protein and vitamins, to help seniors stay healthy. The ingredients used are also high in antioxidants, which can help reduce inflammation and improve cognitive function. Whether you are cooking for a family member or a loved one, these recipes can help make meals both tasty and beneficial.

These recipes are also tailored to meet the needs of seniors with Alzheimer's disease, meaning they are lower in fat and sodium content, and free of added sugar. Additionally, they are designed to be served in smaller portions, so seniors feel satisfied without overindulging. Furthermore, the recipes are also designed to be easy to remember, so that seniors can follow the instructions with minimal assistance. With these recipes, seniors will be able to enjoy delicious and nutritious meals, while also providing them with the necessary nutrients and health benefits that they need.

Let's go ahead to list recipes for breakfast, lunch, dinner, snacks, and desserts. These recipes would also include instructions on how to create these meals with ease.

Breakfast Recipes

1. Egg and Cheese Toast

Ingredients:

- 2 slices of whole grain bread
- 1 egg
- 1 slice of cheese

Instructions:

- Toast the bread until golden brown
- Heat a nonstick skillet over medium heat
- Crack the egg into the pan and scramble until cooked
- Place the scrambled egg onto one slice of the toast
- Place the cheese on top of the egg
- Top with the other toast slice
- Serve warm

Time: 10 minutes

2. Overnight Oats

Ingredients:

- ½ cup rolled oats
- ½ cup milk
- 1 tablespoon honey
- ¼ cup fresh fruit

Instructions:

- Place the oats, milk, honey and fruit into a mason jar

- Stir until the ingredients are completely combined
- Secure the lid of the jar and place in the fridge overnight
- In the morning, scoop the oats into a bowl and enjoy

Time: 10 minutes (overnight)

3. Fruit Smoothie

Ingredients:
- ½ cup frozen fruit
- ½ cup plain yogurt
- ½ cup milk

Instructions:
- Place the frozen fruit, yogurt and milk into a blender
- Blend until the ingredients are completely smooth
- Serve cold

Time: 5 minutes

4. Avocado Toast

Ingredients:
- 2 slices of whole grain bread
- ½ avocado, 1 teaspoon olive oil

\

Instructions:
- Toast the bread until golden brown
- Slice the avocado in half, remove the pit and scoop out the flesh
- Spread the avocado onto the toast
- Sprinkle the olive oil on top of the avocado
- Serve warm

Time: 5 minutes

5. Yogurt Parfait

Ingredients:
- ½ cup plain yogurt
- ¼ cup granola
- ¼ cup fresh fruit

Instructions:
- Place the yogurt into a bowl
- Top with the granola and fresh fruit and enjoy

Time: 5 minutes

6. Egg Muffins

Ingredients:
- 4 eggs
- ¼ cup shredded cheese
- ¼ cup diced vegetables

Instructions:
- Preheat the oven to 350 degrees
- Grease a muffin tin with nonstick cooking spray
- Crack the eggs into a bowl and whisk until mixed
- Stir in the cheese and vegetables
- Evenly distribute the mixture among the muffin cups.
- Bake for 15 minutes or until the eggs are set
- Serve warm

Time: 20 minutes

7. French Toast

Ingredients:

- 2 slices of whole grain bread
- 2 eggs
- 2 tablespoons milk

Instructions:

- Place the bread slices into a shallow dish
- Whisk the eggs and milk together in a another bowl.
- Pour the egg mixture over the bread slices, flipping to coat both sides
- A nonstick skillet should be heated to medium.
- Add the bread slices and cook until golden brown
- Serve warm with desired toppings

Time: 10 minutes

8. Banana Oat Pancakes

Ingredients:

- 1 ripe banana
- ½ cup rolled oats
- ½ teaspoon baking powder
- 1 egg

Instructions:

- Place the banana, oats, baking powder and egg into a blender
- Blend until the ingredients are completely combined
- Heat a nonstick skillet over medium heat

- Grease the pan with nonstick cooking spray
- Scoop 1/4 cup of the batter onto the skillet and cook until golden brown
- Cook the opposite side until golden brown after flipping.
- Serve warm with desired toppings

Time: 10 minutes

9. Ham and Cheese Sandwich

Ingredients:
- 2 slices of whole grain bread
- 2 slices of ham
- 1 slice of cheese

Instructions:
- Toast the bread until golden brown
- Place the ham and cheese onto one slice of the toast
- Top with the other toast slice
- Serve warm

Time: 5 minutes

10. Oatmeal

Ingredients:
- ½ cup rolled oats
- 1 cup milk
- 1 tablespoon honey

Instructions:
- Place the oats, milk and honey into a small saucepan
- Heat over medium heat and stir until the oats are cooked
- Serve warm with desired toppings

Time: 10 minutes

11. Soft Boiled Eggs

Ingredients:
- 2 eggs
- 2 tablespoons butter
- Salt and pepper to taste

Instructions:
- Bring a medium saucepan to a boil over a full pot of water.
- Carefully lower the eggs into the boiling water and let cook for 6 minutes
- Remove the eggs from the pan and place in a bowl of ice water for 1 minute
- Peel and serve with buttered toast and salt and pepper to taste

Time: 10 minutes

12. Banana Pancakes

Ingredients:
- 1 cup all-purpose flour
- 2 tablespoons sugar
- 2 teaspoons baking powder
- ½ teaspoon salt
- 1 cup milk

- 1 large banana, mashed
- 2 tablespoons vegetable oil

Instructions:
- Combine the flour, sugar, baking soda, and salt in a big bowl.
- In a separate bowl, mix together the milk, mashed banana, and oil.
- Just combine the dry ingredients with the addition of the wet ingredients.
- Heat a skillet or griddle over medium heat and grease with butter or oil.
- Drop the pancake batter by 1/4 cupfuls onto the skillet and cook until bubbles start to form, about 2 minutes.
- Flip the pancakes and cook for an additional 1-2 minutes.
- Serve with desired toppings.

Time: 15 minutes

13. Avocado Toast

Ingredients:
- 2 slices of bread
- ½ ripe avocado
- 1 teaspoon olive oil
- Salt and pepper to taste

Instructions:
- Toast the bread until golden brown.
- Mash the avocado in a bowl and stir in the olive oil, salt, and pepper.
- Spread the mashed avocado onto the toast and serve.

Time: 5 minutes

14. Savory Breakfast Egg Muffins

Ingredients:
- 5 eggs
- ½ cup diced bell peppers
- ½ cup diced mushrooms
- ¼ cup diced onions
- ¼ cup shredded gruyere cheese
- Salt and pepper to taste.

Instructions:
- Preheat the oven to 375°F.
- Grease a 12-cup muffin tin.
- In a bowl, whisk together the eggs, bell peppers, mushrooms, onions, and cheese.
- Divide the mixture evenly among the muffin cups, adding salt and pepper to taste.
- Bake for 20 minutes.

Time: 25 minutes

15. Peanut Butter and Banana Toast

Ingredients:

- 2 slices whole wheat bread
- 2 tablespoons peanut butter
- 1 banana, sliced
- 1 teaspoon honey

Instructions:

- Toast the bread.
- Spread the peanut butter on each slice.
- Top with the sliced banana and drizzle with honey.

Time: 5 minutes

16. Blueberry Oat Smoothie

Ingredients:

- ½ cup plain Greek yogurt,
- ½ cup skim milk,
- ½ cup frozen blueberries,
- ½ cup rolled oats,
- 1 tablespoon agave syrup.

Instructions:

- Place all the ingredients in a blender and blend until smooth.
- Pour into a glass and enjoy.

Time: 5 minutes

17. Egg and Cheese Breakfast Burrito

Ingredients:

- 2 eggs, scrambled
- 2 tablespoons diced tomatoes
- 2 tablespoons diced onions
- 2 tablespoons diced bell peppers
- 2 tablespoons shredded cheddar cheese
- 2 tablespoons salsa
- 1 whole wheat tortilla.

Instructions:

- Place the scrambled eggs, tomatoes, onions, bell peppers, and cheese in the center of the tortilla.
- Top with salsa and fold the tortilla over the filling.
- Heat a non-stick skillet over medium heat and cook the burrito for 2 minutes per side, until the cheese is melted and the tortilla is lightly browned.

Time: 10 minutes

18. Baked Oatmeal

Ingredients:

- 2 cups rolled oats
- 2 cups skim milk
- 1 teaspoon ground cinnamon
- 1 teaspoon ground nutmeg
- 2 tablespoons brown sugar
- ¼ cup raisins.

Instructions:
- Preheat the oven to 350°F.
- In a bowl, combine the oats, milk, cinnamon, nutmeg, and brown sugar.
- Spread the mixture into a greased 9x13-inch baking dish and sprinkle with the raisins.
- Bake for 40 minutes.

Time: 45 minutes

19. Vegetable Omelet

Ingredients:
- 2 eggs, beaten
- 2 tablespoons diced tomatoes
- 2 tablespoons diced bell peppers
- 2 tablespoons diced onions
- 2 tablespoons shredded cheddar cheese
- Salt and pepper to taste.

Instructions:
- Heat a non-stick skillet over medium heat.
- Add the beaten eggs to the skillet and cook for 1 minute.
- Add the tomatoes, bell peppers, and onions and cook for an additional 2 minutes, stirring occasionally.
- Top with the cheese and season with salt and pepper to taste.
- Fold the omelet in half and cook for an additional 3 minutes.

Time: 10 minutes

20. Whole Grain Cereal with Fruits

Ingredients:

- 1 cup whole grain cereal (oatmeal or wheat flakes)
- 1 cup skim milk
- ½ cup fresh berries
- 1 tablespoon honey.

Instructions:

- Place the cereal and milk in a bowl and mix together.
- Top with the fresh berries and drizzle with honey.

Time: 5 minutes

21. Protein Berry Breakfast Bowl

Ingredients:

- ½ cup plain Greek yogurt
- ¼ cup toasted almonds
- ¼ cup chopped walnuts
- 1 cup fresh berries
- 1 teaspoon honey
- ½ teaspoon ground cinnamon

Instructions:

- Place the yogurt in a bowl and top with the almonds, walnuts, berries, honey, and cinnamon.

Time: 5 minutes

22. Baked Egg and Cheese

Ingredients:

- 2 eggs,
- 2 tablespoons shredded cheddar cheese,
- 2 tablespoons diced tomatoes,
- 2 tablespoons diced bell peppers,
- 2 tablespoons diced onions.

Instructions:

- Preheat the oven to 375°F.
- Grease a 9x13-inch baking dish.
- Place the eggs in the dish and top with the cheese, tomatoes, bell peppers, and onions.
- Bake for 20 minutes.

Time: 25 minutes

23. Turkey Bacon and Egg Sandwich

Ingredients:

- 2 slices whole wheat bread
- 2 slices turkey bacon, cooked
- 1 egg, scrambled
- 1 tablespoon light mayonnaise.

Instructions:

- Toast the bread.
- Top one slice of bread with the turkey bacon and scrambled egg.

- Spread the mayonnaise on the other slice of bread and place it on top.

Time: 5 minutes

24. Egg and Cheese Breakfast Wrap

Ingredients:
- 1 whole wheat tortilla
- 2 eggs, scrambled
- tablespoons shredded cheddar cheese
- 2 tablespoons salsa.

Instructions:
- Place the scrambled eggs, cheese, and salsa in the center of the tortilla.
- Fold the sides of the tortilla over the filling and serve.

Time: 5 minutes

25. Chia Seed Pudding

Ingredients:
- ¼ cup chia seeds
- 1 cup skim milk
- 1 teaspoon honey

Instructions:
- Place the chia seeds and milk in a bowl and mix together.
- Cover and refrigerate for at least 4 hours, or overnight.
- Stir in the honey before serving.

Time: 4 hours (overnight)

26. Omelet Bites

Ingredients:

- 5 eggs, beaten
- 2 tablespoons diced tomatoes
- 2 tablespoons diced bell peppers
- 2 tablespoons diced onions
- 2 tablespoons shredded cheddar cheese
- Salt and pepper to taste

Instructions:

- Preheat the oven to 375°F.
- Grease a 12-cup muffin tin.
- In a bowl, whisk together the eggs, tomatoes, bell peppers, onions, and cheese.
- Divide the mixture evenly among the muffin cups, adding salt and pepper to taste.
- Bake for 20 minutes.

Time: 25 minutes

27. Tofu Scramble

Ingredients:

- 1 package firm tofu, crumbled
- 2 tablespoons olive oil
- 2 tablespoons diced tomatoes
- 2 tablespoons diced bell peppers
- 2 tablespoons diced onions
- Salt and pepper to taste.

Instructions:
- Heat the olive oil in a non-stick skillet over medium heat.
- Add the crumbled tofu and cook for 5 minutes.
- Add the tomatoes, bell peppers, and onions and cook for an additional 5 minutes, stirring occasionally.
- Season with salt and pepper to taste.

Time: 10 minutes

28. Overnight Oats

Ingredients:
- ½ cup rolled oats
- ½ cup skim milk
- 1 teaspoon honey
- 1 tablespoon chia seeds.

Instructions:
- Place the oats, milk, honey, and chia seeds in a jar and stir together.
- Cover and refrigerate overnight.

Time: 5 minutes (plus overnight)

29. Egg and Avocado Toast

Ingredients:
- 2 slices whole wheat bread
- 2 eggs, fried
- ½ an avocado, mashed
- Salt and pepper to taste.

Instructions:
- Toast the bread.
- Top each slice with a fried egg and mashed avocado.
- Season with salt and pepper to taste.

Time: 10 minutes

30. Breakfast Burrito

Ingredients:
- 2 eggs, scrambled
- 2 tablespoons shredded cheddar cheese
- 2 tablespoons diced tomatoes
- 2 tablespoons diced bell peppers
- 2 tablespoons diced onions
- 2 tablespoons salsa
- 2 whole wheat tortillas.

Instructions:
- A nonstick skillet should be heated to medium.
- Add the eggs, cheese, tomatoes, bell peppers, and onions and cook for 3 minutes, stirring occasionally.
- Place the mixture in the center of the tortillas and top with salsa.
- Serve the tortillas by folding the edges over the contents.

Time: 10 minutes

Lunch Recipes.

1. Ham and Cheese Panini

Ingredients:
- 2 slices of whole grain bread
- 2 slices of ham
- 2 slices of cheddar cheese
- 2 tablespoons of butter
- 1 teaspoon of olive oil

Instructions:
- Heat butter and olive oil in a skillet over medium-high heat.
- Place bread slices in the skillet and layer ham and cheese on one slice.
- Place the other piece of bread on top and press down softly.
- /Cook for 3-4 minutes per side until golden brown and cheese is melted.

Time: 10 minutes

2. Tuna Salad Sandwich

Ingredients:
- 2 cans of tuna
- ¼ cup of celery
- 1/4 cup of onion
- 2 tablespoons of mayonnaise
- 1 teaspoon of mustard
- 2 tablespoons of relish

- 8 slices of whole grain bread

Instructions:

- Drain tuna and place in a bowl.
- Add celery, onion, mayonnaise, mustard, and relish and mix together until combined.
- Spread tuna salad onto 4 slices of bread and top with remaining bread slices.
- Cut sandwiches in half and serve.

Time: 10 minutes

3. Egg Salad Sandwich

Ingredients:

- 6 eggs
- ¼ cup of mayonnaise
- 1 teaspoon of mustard
- 1 tablespoon of relish
- 10 slices of whole grain bread

Instructions:

- Boil eggs for 8-10 minutes.
- Peel eggs and place in a bowl.
- Mash eggs and add mayonnaise, mustard, and relish. Mix until combined.
- Spread egg salad onto 5 slices of bread and top with remaining bread slices.
- Cut sandwiches in half and serve.

Time: 15 minutes

4. Turkey and Cheese Wrap:

Ingredients:

- 2 tablespoons of cream cheese
- ¼ cup of shredded cheddar cheese
- 2 tablespoons of chopped green onion
- 2 tablespoons of diced red pepper
- ¼ teaspoon of garlic powder
- ¼ teaspoon of paprika
- 4 large flour tortillas
- 8 ounces of deli sliced turkey

Instructions:

- In a bowl, mix together cream cheese, cheddar cheese, green onion, red pepper, garlic powder, and paprika.
- Spread cheese mixture onto the tortillas and top with turkey slices.
- Wrap tortillas and cut in half and serve.

Time: 10 minutes

5. Grilled Cheese and Tomato Soup

Ingredients:

- 2 tablespoons of butter
- 2 slices of whole grain bread
- 2 slices of cheddar cheese
- 1 can of tomato soup

Instructions:
- Heat butter in a skillet over medium-high heat.
- Place bread slices in the skillet and layer cheese on one slice.
- Lay the other slice of bread on top and press down softly.
- Cook for 3-4 minutes per side until golden brown and cheese is melted.
- Heat soup in a pot over medium heat until warmed through.
- Serve with grilled cheese.

Time: 10 minutes

6. Chicken Quesadilla:

Ingredients:
- 2 tablespoons of butter
- 2 large flour tortillas
- ½ cup of cooked chicken
- ¼ cup of black beans, 1/4 cup of corn
- ¼ cup of shredded cheddar cheese

Instructions:
- Heat butter in a skillet over medium-high heat.
- Place one tortilla in the skillet and layer chicken, black beans, corn, and cheese on top.
- Place the other tortilla on top and press down gently.
- Cook for 3-4 minutes per side until golden brown and cheese is melted.
- Cut quesadilla in half and serve.

Time: 10 minutes

7. Avocado Toast

Ingredients:
- 2 slices of whole grain bread
- ½ avocado
- ¼ teaspoon of garlic powder
- ¼ teaspoon of smoked paprika
- ¼ teaspoon of black pepper

Instructions:
- Toast bread slices in a toaster.
- Mash avocado in a bowl and mix in garlic powder, smoked paprika, and black pepper.
- Spread avocado mixture onto toast and serve.

Time: 5 minutes

8. Peanut Butter and Banana Sandwich

Ingredients:
- 2 tablespoons of peanut butter
- 1 banana
- 2 slices of whole grain bread

Instructions:
- Spread peanut butter onto one slice of bread and top with sliced banana.
- Place the other slice of bread on top and press down lightly.
- Cut sandwich in half and serve.

Time: 5 minutes

9. Greek Yogurt Parfait

Ingredients:

- 1 cup of plain Greek yogurt
- ¼ cup of granola
- ¼ cup of fresh blueberries

Instructions:

- Layer yogurt, granola, and blueberries in a bowl.
- Serve.

Time: 5 minutes

10. Cheese and Cracker Plate

Ingredients:

- 4 slices of cheddar cheese
- 4 slices of Swiss cheese
- 8 whole wheat crackers

Instructions:

- Place cheese and crackers on a plate. Serve.

Time: 5 minutes

11. Peanut Butter and Banana Sandwiches

Ingredients:

- 2 slices of whole wheat bread
- 2 tablespoons of peanut butter
- 1 banana

Instructions:
- Spread the peanut butter on each slice of bread.
- Slice the banana and place on one slice of bread.
- Place the other slice of bread on top and cut into halves. Serve.

Time: 10 minutes

12. Egg Salad Wraps
Ingredients:
- 2 hard boiled eggs
- 2 tablespoons of mayonnaise
- 2 whole wheat tortillas
- 2 leaves of lettuce

Instructions:
- Mash the hard boiled eggs and mix with mayonnaise.
- Spread the egg salad onto the tortillas and top with lettuce.
- Roll up the tortillas and cut in half. Serve.

Time: 10 minutes

13. Tomato Soup and Grilled Cheese
Ingredients:
- 1 can of tomato soup
- 2 slices of whole wheat bread
- 2 slices of cheddar cheese

Instructions:
- Heat the tomato soup in a pot. Meanwhile, heat a pan over medium heat.

- Place the cheese between two slices of bread and cook until the cheese is melted and the bread is golden brown.
- Serve the soup with the grilled cheese.

Time: 15 minutes

14. Chickpea and Avocado Salad

Ingredients:
- ½ cup of cooked chickpeas
- ¼ cup of diced tomatoes
- ¼ cup of diced cucumber
- ¼ cup of diced red onion
- ½ an avocado
- 2 tablespoons of olive oil
- 1 tablespoon of white wine vinegar

Instructions:
- Place the chickpeas, tomatoes, cucumber, and red onion in a bowl.
- Slice the avocado in half, remove the pit, and dice.
- Add the avocado to the bowl.
- Drizzle with olive oil and white wine vinegar.
- Toss to combine. Serve.

Time: 10 minutes

15. Tuna Salad Sandwich

Ingredients:

- 1 can of tuna
- 2 tablespoons of mayonnaise
- 2 slices of whole wheat bread
- 1 lettuce leaf

Instructions:

- Drain the tuna and place in a bowl.
- Add the mayonnaise and mix to combine.
- Spread the tuna salad onto the slices of bread and top with the lettuce leaf.
- Place the other slice of bread on top.
- Cut into halves and serve.

Time: 10 minutes

16. Turkey and Cucumber Roll-Ups

Ingredients:

- 4 slices of deli turkey
- ½ cucumber
- 1 tablespoon of cream cheese

Instructions:

- Spread the cream cheese onto each slice of turkey.
- Slice the cucumber into thin strips and place on top of the cream cheese.
- Roll up the slices of turkey and cut into halves. Serve.

Time: 10 minutes

17. Hummus and Veggies

Ingredients:

- ½ cup of prepared hummus
- ½ cup of sliced carrots
- ½ cup of sliced celery
- ½ cup of bell pepper slices

Instructions:

- Place the hummus in a bowl and top with the vegetables. Serve.

Time: 5 minutes

18. Apple and Peanut Butter

Ingredients:

- 1 apple
- 2 tablespoons of peanut butter

Instructions:

- Cut the apple into slices.
- Spread the peanut butter onto each slice. Serve.

Time: 5 minutes

19. Quesadilla

Ingredients:

- 2 whole wheat tortillas
- ¼ cup of shredded cheddar cheese

Instructions:
- Place one tortilla in a pan over medium heat.
- Sprinkle the cheese onto the tortilla and top with the other tortilla.
- Cook for 2-3 minutes or until the cheese is melted and the tortilla is golden brown.
- Cut into halves and serve.

Time: 10 minutes

20. Fruit Salad

Ingredients:
- ½ cup of diced apples
- ½ cup of diced oranges
- ½ cup of diced strawberries
- 2 tablespoons of honey

Instructions:
- Place the apples, oranges, and strawberries in a bowl.
- Drizzle with honey and mix to combine. Serve.

Time: 5 minutes

21. Baked Salmon

Ingredients:
- 4 salmon fillets
- 2 tablespoons of olive oil
- 1 teaspoon of salt
- ¼ teaspoon of pepper

Instructions:
- Preheat oven to 400°F.
- Place salmon on a baking sheet and season with salt and pepper.
- Drizzle with olive oil.
- Bake for 10-15 minutes or until salmon is cooked through. Serve.

Time: 15 minutes

22. Macaroni and Cheese

Ingredients:
- 2 cups of elbow macaroni
- ¼ cup of butter
- ¼ cup of all-purpose flour
- 2 cups of milk
- ½ cup of shredded cheddar cheese

Instructions:
- Cook the macaroni according to package instructions.
- In a saucepan over medium-low heat, melt the butter.
- Add the flour and whisk to combine.
- Slowly add the milk and whip until thickened.
- Add the cheese and stir until melted.
- Add the cooked macaroni and stir to combine. Serve.

Time: 15 minutes

23. Chicken Soup

Ingredients:

- 2 tablespoons of olive oil
- 1 onion, diced
- 2 carrots, diced
- 2 celery stalks, diced
- 2 cloves of garlic, minced
- 4 cups of chicken broth
- 2 cups of shredded cooked chicken

Instructions:

- Heat the olive oil in a big pot over medium heat.
- Add the onion, carrots, celery, and garlic and simmer for 5 minutes.
- Add the chicken broth and bring the soup to a boil.
- Add the chicken and adjust the heat to low.
- Simmer for 10 minutes. Serve.

Time: 15 minutes

24. Grilled Cheese

Ingredients:

- 2 slices of bread
- 1 tablespoon of butter
- 2 slices of cheese

Instructions:

- Heat a skillet over medium heat.
- Spread the butter on one side of each slice of bread.

- Place one slice of bread in the skillet, butter side down.
- Top with a piece of cheese and the other slice of bread, butter side up.
- Cook for 2-3 minutes or until the cheese is melted and the bread is golden brown. Serve.

Time: 5 minutes

25. Peanut Butter and Banana Sandwich

Ingredients:
- 2 slices of bread
- 2 tablespoons of peanut butter
- 1 banana, sliced

Instructions:
- Spread the peanut butter on one side of each slice of bread.
- Top one slice of bread with the banana slices.
- Top with the other slice of bread.
- Cut in half and serve.

Time: 5 minutes

26. Omelette

Ingredients:
- 2 eggs
- 2 tablespoons of milk
- 1 tablespoon of butter
- ¼ cup of diced vegetables (optional)

Instructions:
- In a bowl, whisk the eggs and milk together.
- Heat the butter in a skillet over medium heat.
- Pour the egg mixture into the skillet.
- If desired, add the vegetables.
- Cook until the eggs are set.
- Flip and cook for 1-2 minutes. Serve.

Time: 10 minutes

27. Cheese and Crackers

Ingredients:
- 4 crackers
- 2 slices of cheese

Instructions:
- Place the crackers on a plate.
- Top each cracker with a slice of cheese. Serve.

Time: 5 minutes

28. Yogurt Parfait

Ingredients:
- 1 cup of plain Greek yogurt
- ¼ cup of granola
- ¼ cup of fresh berries

Instructions:
- Place the yogurt in a bowl.
- Top with the granola and berries. Serve.

Time: 5 minutes

29. Tuna Salad Sandwich

Ingredients:
- 2 slices of bread
- ½ cup of canned tuna
- 2 tablespoons of mayonnaise
- 2 slices of cheese

Instructions:
- In a bowl, combine the tuna and mayonnaise.
- Spread the tuna mixture on one slice of bread.
- Top with the cheese and the other slice of bread.
- Cut in half and serve.

Time: 10 minutes

30. Egg Salad Sandwich

Ingredients:
- 2 slices of bread
- 2 hard-boiled eggs
- 2 tablespoons of mayonnaise

Instructions:
- Mash the eggs in a bowl.
- Add the mayonnaise and mix to combine.
- Spread the egg mixture on one slice of bread.
- Top with the other slice of bread.
- Cut in half and serve.

Time: 10 minutes

Dinner recipes.

1. Baked Salmon with Herbs

Ingredients:
- 4 salmon filets
- 2 tablespoons olive oil,
- 2 tablespoons butter,
- 2 tablespoons chopped fresh parsley
- 2 tablespoons fresh lemon juice
- 1 teaspoon fresh thyme leaves
- 1 teaspoon salt
- ½ teaspoon black pepper

Instructions:
- Preheat oven to 350 degrees F.
- In a small bowl, mix together the olive oil, butter, parsley, lemon juice, thyme leaves, salt and pepper.
- Place the salmon filets in a baking dish and spread the olive oil mixture over them.
- Bake for 15 minutes, or until fish is cooked through.

Time: 15 minutes

2. Vegetable Stir-Fry

Ingredients:
- 2 tablespoons olive oil
- 2 cloves garlic, minced
- 1 red bell pepper, sliced

- 1 green bell pepper, sliced
- 1 red onion, sliced
- 1 cup broccoli florets
- 1 cup sliced mushrooms
- 2 tablespoons soy sauce
- 2 tablespoons honey

Instructions:

- Heat the olive oil in a large skillet over medium-high heat.
- Add the garlic, bell peppers, onion and broccoli.
- Stir-fry for 4 minutes, or until vegetables are barely tender.
- Add the mushrooms and stir-fry for an additional 2 minutes.
- Add the soy sauce and honey and stir-fry for 1 minute.
- Serve hot.

Time: 10 minutes

3. Chicken Fajitas

Ingredients:

- 2 tablespoons olive oil
- 1 pound boneless, skinless chicken breasts, cut into strips
- 1 red bell pepper, sliced
- 1 green bell pepper, sliced
- 1 red onion, sliced
- 2 cloves garlic, minced
- 1 teaspoon chili powder
- 1 teaspoon cumin
- 1 teaspoon salt
- ½ teaspoon black pepper

- 8 flour tortillas

Instructions:

- Heat the olive oil in a large skillet over medium-high heat.
- Add the chicken strips, bell peppers, onion, garlic, chili powder, cumin, salt and pepper.
- Cook for 8 minutes, stirring occasionally, until the chicken is cooked through and the vegetables are tender.
- Warm the tortillas in the microwave for 30 seconds.
- Serve the chicken and vegetables in the tortillas.

Time: 15 minutes

4. Egg Fried Rice

Ingredients:

- 2 tablespoons olive oil
- 2 cloves garlic, minced
- 2 cups cooked white rice
- 2 eggs, beaten
- ½ cup frozen peas
- ½ cup diced carrots
- 2 tablespoons soy sauce

Instructions:
- Heat the olive oil in a large skillet over medium heat.
- Add the garlic and cook for 1 minute.
- Add the cooked rice and stir-fry for 3 minutes.
- Add the eggs and cook, stirring, for 2 minutes.
- Add the peas and carrots and stir-fry for 2 minutes.
- Add the soy sauce and stir-fry for 1 minute. Serve hot.

Time: 10 minutes

5. Baked Ziti

Ingredients:
- 1 pound ziti pasta, cooked
- 2 tablespoons olive oil
- 2 cloves garlic, minced
- 1 onion, diced
- 1 (28-ounce) can crushed tomatoes
- 1 teaspoon dried oregano
- ½ teaspoon salt
- ¼ teaspoon black pepper
- 1 cup ricotta cheese
- 1 cup shredded mozzarella cheese

Instructions:
- Preheat oven to 350 degrees F.
- Grease a 9x13-inch baking dish.
- In a large saucepan, heat the olive oil over medium heat.
- Add the garlic and onion and cook for 5 minutes, or until onion is softened.

- Add the crushed tomatoes, oregano, salt and pepper and simmer for 10 minutes.
- In a large bowl, combine the cooked ziti, ricotta cheese, mozzarella cheese and tomato sauce.
- Pour into the prepared baking dish and bake for 30 minutes, or until cheese is melted and bubbly.

Time: 40 minutes

6. Baked Chicken Parmesan

Ingredients:
- 2 boneless, skinless chicken breasts
- ½ cup Italian-style breadcrumbs
- 2 tablespoons olive oil
- ¼ cup grated Parmesan cheese
- ½ teaspoon garlic powder
- ½ teaspoon dried oregano
- ½ teaspoon salt
- ¼ teaspoon black pepper
- ½ cup marinara sauce

Instructions:
- Preheat oven to 375 degrees F.
- Grease a baking sheet with cooking spray.
- In a small bowl, mix the breadcrumbs, Parmesan cheese, garlic powder, oregano, salt and pepper.
- In another small dish, add the olive oil..
- Dip each chicken breast in the olive oil, then in the breadcrumb mixture.

- Arrange the chicken breasts on the prepared baking sheet.
- Bake for 20 minutes, or until chicken is cooked through.
- Top with the marinara sauce and bake for an additional 5 minutes.

Time: 25 minutes

7. Mediterranean Salad

Ingredients:
- 4 cups mixed salad greens
- ½ cup cherry tomatoes, halved
- ½ cup cucumber, diced
- ¼ cup kalamata olives
- ¼ cup feta cheese, crumbled
- 2 tablespoons olive oil
- 1 tablespoon red wine vinegar
- 1 teaspoon honey
- ¼ teaspoon garlic powder
- ¼ teaspoon salt
- ¼ teaspoon black pepper

Instructions:
- In a large bowl, combine the salad greens, cherry tomatoes, cucumber, olives and feta cheese.
- In a small bowl, whisk together the olive oil, red wine vinegar, honey, garlic powder, salt and pepper.
- Drizzle the dressing over the salad and toss to mix.
- Serve immediately.

Time: 10 minutes

8. Lentil Stew

Ingredients:
- 2 tablespoons olive oil
- 1 onion, diced
- 2 cloves garlic, minced
- 2 carrots, diced
- 1 celery stalk, diced
- 1 cup dry lentils
- 2 cups vegetable broth
- 1 teaspoon dried thyme
- ½ teaspoon salt
- ¼ teaspoon black pepper

Instructions:
- Heat the olive oil in a large pot over medium heat.
- Add the onion, garlic, carrots and celery and cook for 5 minutes.
- Add the lentils, vegetable broth, thyme, salt and pepper and bring to a boil.
- Reduce heat to low, cover and simmer for 30 minutes, or until lentils are tender.
- Serve hot.

Time: 35 minutes

9. French Toast

Ingredients:

- 4 slices white bread
- 2 eggs, beaten
- 2 tablespoons milk
- 2 tablespoons melted butter
- ½ teaspoon ground cinnamon
- ¼ teaspoon ground nutmeg
- 2 tablespoons maple syrup

Instructions:

- Preheat a large skillet over medium heat.
- In a shallow bowl, whisk together the eggs, milk, butter, cinnamon and nutmeg.
- Dip each slice of bread in the egg mixture and place in the skillet.
- Cook for 3 minutes per side, or until golden brown.
- Drizzle each slice with maple syrup before serving.

Time: 10 minutes

10. Baked Potatoes

Ingredients:

- 4 large baking potatoes
- 2 tablespoons olive oil
- 1 teaspoon garlic powder
- 1 teaspoon dried oregano
- ½ teaspoon salt
- ¼ teaspoon black pepper

Instructions:
- Preheat oven to 400 degrees F.
- Grease a baking sheet with cooking spray.
- Wash and dry the potatoes.
- Rub the potatoes with the olive oil, then sprinkle with the garlic powder, oregano, salt and pepper.
- Place the potatoes on the prepared baking sheet and bake for 30 minutes, or until potatoes are tender.
- Serve hot.

Time: 35 minutes

11. Baked Fish Fillets

Ingredients:
- 4 white fish fillets
- ¼ cup olive oil
- 1 teaspoon garlic powder
- 1 teaspoon dried oregano
- ½ teaspoon salt
- ¼ teaspoon black pepper

Instructions:
- Preheat oven to 400 degrees F.
- Grease a baking sheet with cooking spray.
- Wash and dry the fish fillets.
- Rub the fish with the olive oil, then sprinkle with the garlic powder, oregano, salt and pepper.
- Place the fillets on the prepared baking sheet and bake for 15 minutes, or until cooked through.
- Serve hot.

Time: 20 minutes

12. Chicken and Rice Soup

Ingredients:
- 2 tablespoons olive oil
- 1 small onion, diced
- 2 cloves garlic, minced
- 2-3 boneless, skinless chicken breasts, cut into cubes
- 2 cups chicken broth
- 1 cup cooked brown rice
- ½ teaspoon salt
- ¼ teaspoon black pepper
- ¼ teaspoon dried thyme

Instructions:
- Heat the olive oil in a large pot over medium heat.
- Add the onion and garlic and cook for about 5 minutes, until softened.

- Add the chicken and cook for about 5 minutes, until lightly browned.
- Add the chicken broth, cooked rice, salt, pepper, and thyme.
- Reduce heat to low and simmer for about 10 minutes.
- Serve hot.

Time: 20 minutes

13. Baked Salmon with Roasted Broccoli

Ingredients:

- 4-6 oz salmon filets
- 2 cups broccoli florets
- 2 tablespoons olive oil
- Salt, pepper, and garlic powder

Instructions:

- Preheat oven to 375°F.
- Place salmon and broccoli on a greased baking dish.
- Drizzle olive oil over the salmon and vegetables.
- Sprinkle seasonings and toss to coat.
- Bake for 20-25 minutes, or until salmon is cooked and vegetables are tender.

Time: 25 minutes

14. Baked Apple Slices

Ingredients:
- 4 apples, cored and sliced
- ¼ cup brown sugar
- 1 teaspoon ground cinnamon
- 2 tablespoons butter

Instructions:
- Preheat oven to 350 degrees F.
- Grease a baking dish with cooking spray.
- Place the apple slices in the baking dish.
- In a small bowl, combine the brown sugar and cinnamon.
- Sprinkle the mixture over the apples and dot with the butter.
- Bake for 15 minutes, or until apples are tender. Serve warm.

Time: 20 minutes

15. Vegetable Stir-Fry

Ingredients:
- 2 tablespoons olive oil
- 1 small onion, diced
- 2 cloves garlic, minced
- 2 carrots, sliced
- 1 red bell pepper, diced
- 1 cup broccoli florets
- 1 cup cooked brown rice
- 2 tablespoons soy sauce

Instructions:
- Heat the oil in a large skillet over medium heat.
- Add the onion and garlic and cook for about 5 minutes.
- Add the carrots, bell pepper, and broccoli and cook for an additional 5 minutes.
- Add the cooked rice and soy sauce and stir to combine.
- Cook for an additional 2 minutes, or until vegetables are tender.
- Serve hot.

Time: 15 minutes

16. Egg and Cheese Frittata

Ingredients:
- 8 eggs
- ¼ cup milk
- ½ teaspoon salt
- ¼ teaspoon black pepper
- 1 cup shredded cheddar cheese
- ½ cup diced ham

Instructions:
- Preheat oven to 375 degrees F.
- Grease an 8-inch baking dish with cooking spray.
- In a large bowl, whisk together the eggs, milk, salt and pepper.
- Add the cheese and ham and stir to combine.
- Pour the mixture into the prepared baking dish and bake for 25 minutes, or until eggs are set. Serve hot.

Time: 30 minutes

17. Macaroni and Cheese

Ingredients:

- 1 pound elbow macaroni
- 2 tablespoons butter
- 2 tablespoons all-purpose flour
- 2 cups milk, 1 teaspoon salt
- ¼ teaspoon black pepper
- 2 cups shredded cheddar cheese

Instructions:

- Preheat oven to 350 degrees F.
- Grease a 9x13 inch baking dish with cooking spray.
- Cook the macaroni according to package directions.
- Drain and set aside.
- Melt the butter in a large pot over medium heat.
- Add the flour and whisk for about 1 minute.
- Slowly add the milk, whisking continuously until mixture is smooth.
- Add the salt and pepper and stir in the cheese until melted.
- Add the cooked macaroni and stir to combine.
- Pour the mixture into the prepared baking dish and bake for 20 minutes, or until cheese is bubbly.
- Serve hot.

Time: 30 minutes

18. Baked Sweet Potatoes

Ingredients:
- 4 large sweet potatoes
- 2 tablespoons olive oil
- 1 teaspoon garlic powder
- 1 teaspoon dried oregano
- ½ teaspoon salt
- ¼ teaspoon black pepper

Instructions:
- Preheat oven to 400 degrees F.
- Grease a baking sheet with cooking spray.
- Wash and dry the sweet potatoes.
- Rub the potatoes with the olive oil, then sprinkle with the garlic powder, oregano, salt and pepper.
- Place the potatoes on the prepared baking sheet and bake for 30 minutes, or until potatoes are tender.
- Serve hot.

Time: 35 minutes

19. Chicken and Rice Casserole

Ingredients:
- 2 tablespoons olive oil
- 1 onion, diced
- 2 cloves garlic, minced
- 2 cups cooked chicken, diced
- 2 cups cooked white rice
- 1 teaspoon Italian seasoning

- ½ teaspoon salt
- ¼ teaspoon black pepper
- 2 cups low-sodium chicken broth
- ½ cup shredded mozzarella cheese

Instructions:
- Preheat oven to 375F.
- Grease a 9×13-inch baking dish with cooking spray.
- Heat olive oil in a large skillet over medium heat.
- Add onion and cook until soft and translucent, about 5 minutes.
- Add garlic and cook until fragrant, about 1 minute.
- Add chicken, rice, Italian seasoning, salt and pepper, and cook until heated through, about 3 minutes.
- Transfer mixture to the prepared baking dish and pour chicken broth over the top.
- Sprinkle mozzarella cheese over the top and bake for 25 minutes, or until cheese is melted and bubbly.
- Serve hot.

Time: 30 minutes

20. Creamy Baked Mac and Cheese

Ingredients:
- 4 tablespoons butter
- 4 tablespoons all-purpose flour
- 4 cups milk
- ½ teaspoon garlic powder
- ½ teaspoon onion powder
- 1 teaspoon salt

- ¼ teaspoon black pepper
- 8 ounces elbow macaroni, cooked
- 2 cups sharp cheddar cheese, shredded

Instructions:
- Preheat oven to 350F.
- Grease a 9x13-inch baking dish with cooking spray.
- In a large saucepan, melt butter over medium heat.
- Add flour and whisk together until combined.
- Gradually add milk and whisk until mixture is smooth.
- Add garlic powder, onion powder, salt and pepper and stir to combine.
- Bring mixture to a boil, reduce heat to low and simmer for 5 minutes, stirring occasionally.
- Remove from heat and add cooked macaroni and cheddar cheese and stir to combine.
- Pour macaroni mixture into the prepared baking dish.
- Bake for 25 minutes, or until cheese is melted and bubbly.
- Serve hot.

Time: 35 minutes

21. Stuffed Peppers

Ingredients:
- 4 bell peppers
- 1 tablespoon olive oil
- 1 onion, diced
- 1 cup cooked quinoa
- 1 teaspoon garlic powder

- 1 teaspoon dried oregano
- ½ teaspoon salt
- ¼ teaspoon black pepper
- 1 cup Marinara sauce

Instructions:
- Preheat oven to 375F.
- Grease a 9x13-inch baking dish with cooking spray.
- Cut peppers in half lengthwise and remove the stems and seeds.
- Place peppers in the prepared baking dish. Heat oil in a large skillet over medium heat.
- Add onion and cook until soft and translucent, about 5 minutes.
- Add quinoa, garlic powder, oregano, salt and pepper and cook until heated through, about 3 minutes.
- Remove from heat and stir in Marinara sauce.
- Spoon quinoa mixture into pepper halves.
- Bake for 25 minutes, or until peppers are tender. Serve hot.

Time: 30 minutes

22. Fish and Veggies

Ingredients:
- 1 tablespoon olive oil
- 1 onion, diced
- 2 cloves garlic, minced
- 1 pound white fish, cut into cubes
- 1 teaspoon Italian seasoning
- ½ teaspoon salt
- ¼ teaspoon black pepper

- 2 cups mixed vegetables

Instructions:
- Heat oil in a large skillet over medium heat.
- Add onion and cook until soft and translucent, about 5 minutes.
- Add garlic and cook until fragrant, about 1 minute.
- Add fish, Italian seasoning, salt and pepper and cook until fish is cooked through, about 5 minutes.
- Add vegetables and cook until vegetables are tender, about 5 minutes. Serve hot.

Time: 15 minutes

23. Spinach and Cheese Frittata

Ingredients:
- 4 tablespoons butter
- 1 onion, diced
- 2 cloves garlic, minced
- 4 cups spinach
- ½ teaspoon salt
- ¼ teaspoon black pepper
- 8 eggs
- 1 cup shredded cheddar cheese

Instructions:
- Preheat oven to 375F.
- Grease a 9-inch pie plate with cooking spray.
- Heat butter in a large skillet over medium heat.
- Add onion and cook until soft and translucent, about 5 minutes.

- Add garlic and cook until fragrant, about 1 minute.
- Add spinach and season with salt and pepper.
- Cook until spinach is wilted, about 3 minutes. Remove from heat and set aside.
- In a large bowl, whisk together eggs and cheese until combined.
- Pour egg mixture into the prepared pie plate.
- Top with spinach mixture and spread evenly.
- Bake for 25 minutes, or until eggs are set. Serve hot.

Time: 30 minutes

24. Zucchini and Tomato Bake

Ingredients:
- 2 tablespoons olive oil
- 1 onion, diced
- 2 cloves garlic, minced
- 2 zucchini, sliced
- 1 teaspoon Italian seasoning
- ½ teaspoon salt
- ¼ teaspoon black pepper
- 2 cups diced tomatoes

Instructions:
- Preheat oven to 375F. Grease a 9x13-inch baking dish with cooking spray.
- Heat olive oil in a large skillet over medium heat.
- Add onion and cook until soft and translucent, about 5 minutes.
- Add garlic and cook until fragrant, about 1 minute.

- Add zucchini, Italian seasoning, salt and pepper and cook until zucchini is tender, about 5 minutes.
- Remove from heat and stir in tomatoes.
- Pour vegetable mixture into the prepared baking dish and bake for 20 minutes, or until vegetables are tender. Serve hot.

Time: 25 minutes

25. Stuffed Peppers

Ingredients:
- 4 bell peppers
- 1 teaspoon olive oil
- 1 onion, diced
- 1 clove garlic, minced
- 1 cup cooked quinoa
- ½ cup frozen corn
- ½ cup black beans
- ¼ cup salsa
- ½ teaspoon cumin
- ¼ teaspoon salt
- ¼ teaspoon black pepper

Instructions:
- Preheat oven to 375F.
- Cut the tops off of the bell peppers and remove the seeds.
- Place peppers in a baking dish.
- Heat olive oil in a large skillet over medium heat.
- Add onion and cook until soft and translucent, about 5 minutes.
- Add garlic and cook until fragrant, about 1 minute.

- Add quinoa, corn, black beans, salsa, cumin, salt and pepper and cook for another 5 minutes, stirring occasionally.
- Fill each bell pepper with the quinoa mixture.
- Bake for 20 minutes, or until peppers are tender. Serve hot.

Time: 30 minutes

26. Turkey Wraps

Ingredients:

- 4 large whole wheat tortillas
- 2 tablespoons pesto
- 8 ounces cooked turkey, sliced
- ½ red bell pepper, sliced
- ½ cup shredded lettuce

Instructions:

- Spread each tortilla with pesto.
- Top with turkey, bell pepper and lettuce.
- Roll up the wraps and serve.

Time: 10 minutes

27. Baked Salmon with Asparagus

Ingredients:

- 2 salmon fillets
- 1 tablespoon olive oil
- Salt and pepper to taste
- 2 tablespoons butter,
- 2 cloves garlic, minced
- ½ teaspoon dried oregano

- ½ teaspoon dried thyme
- ½ lemon, thinly sliced
- 6-8 spears asparagus, trimmed

Instructions:
- Preheat oven to 375°F.
- Place salmon on a greased baking sheet and brush with olive oil.
- Sprinkle with salt and pepper.
- Bake for 10-12 minutes, or until cooked through. Meanwhile, melt butter in a large skillet over medium heat.
- Add garlic, oregano, and thyme, and cook until fragrant, about 1 minute.
- Add lemon slices and asparagus and cook until asparagus is just tender, about 4 minutes.
- Place cooked salmon on a serving plate and top with asparagus and lemon slices. Serve warm.

Time: 20 minutes

28. Broccoli and Cheese Frittata

Ingredients:
- 2 tablespoons olive oil
- 1 onion, diced
- 2 cloves garlic, minced
- 2 cups broccoli florets
- 3 eggs, lightly beaten
- ½ cup shredded cheddar cheese
- Salt and pepper to taste

Instructions:
- Heat olive oil in a large oven-proof skillet over medium heat.
- Add onion and cook until soft and translucent, about 5 minutes.
- Add garlic and cook until fragrant, about 1 minute.
- Add broccoli and stir to combine.
- Pour eggs into the skillet and cook until edges are set, about 5 minutes.
- Sprinkle cheese over top and season with salt and pepper.
- Place skillet in preheated oven and bake for 10 minutes, or until eggs are cooked through. Serve warm.

Time: 20 minutes

29. Creamy Macaroni and Cheese

Ingredients:
- 2 cups macaroni (cooked according to package instructions)
- 2 tablespoons butter
- 2 tablespoons all-purpose flour
- 1½ cups milk
- 1/2 cup shredded cheddar cheese
- Salt and pepper to taste

Instructions:
- Preheat oven to 350°F.
- Melt butter in a medium saucepan over medium heat.
- Add flour and whisk to combine.
- Gradually whisk in milk and cook until mixture is thick and bubbly.
- Add cheese and stir until melted.

- Season with salt and pepper.
- Pour cheese sauce over cooked macaroni and stir to combine.
- Transfer to a greased baking dish and bake for 20 minutes, or until bubbly and golden brown. Serve warm.

Time: 30 minutes

30. Beef and Mushroom Stew

Ingredients:
- 2 tablespoons olive oil
- 1 onion, diced
- 2 cloves garlic, minced
- 1½ pounds stew beef, cut into 1-inch cubes
- 8 ounces mushrooms, sliced
- 1 (14.5 ounce) can diced tomatoes
- 1 (14.5 ounce) can beef broth
- 2 tablespoons Worcestershire sauce
- 2 tablespoons tomato paste
- Salt and pepper to taste

Instructions:
- Heat olive oil in a large pot over medium heat.
- Add onion and cook until soft and translucent, about 5 minutes.
- Add garlic and cook until fragrant, about 1 minute.
- Add beef and cook until browned, about 5 minutes.
- Add mushrooms, tomatoes, beef broth, Worcestershire sauce, and tomato paste and stir to combine.

- Bring to a boil, reduce heat, and simmer for 45 minutes, or until beef is tender.
- Season with salt and pepper. Serve hot.

Time: 50 minutes

Snack and Dessert Recipes.

1. Oatmeal Raisin Cookies

Ingredients:
- 2 ½ cups all-purpose flour
- 1 teaspoon baking soda
- 1 teaspoon salt
- 1 cup butter, softened
- ½ cup white sugar
- ½ cup packed light brown sugar
- 2 eggs
- 1 teaspoon vanilla extract
- 2 cups quick-cooking oats
- ½ cup raisins

Instructions:
- Preheat the oven to 375 degrees Fahrenheit.
- In a medium bowl, mix together the flour, baking soda and salt.
- In a large bowl, cream together the butter, white sugar and brown sugar until light and fluffy. Beat in the eggs one at a time, then stir in the vanilla.
- Gradually blend in the dry ingredients until just incorporated. Fold in the oats and raisins.
- Drop the dough by teaspoonfuls onto ungreased baking sheets.
- Bake for 8 to 10 minutes in the preheated oven, or until golden brown. Allow cookies to cool on baking sheet for 5 minutes before transferring to a wire rack to cool completely.

Time: 25 minutes

2. Peanut Butter and Jelly Bars

Ingredients:
- 2 cups all-purpose flour
- 1 teaspoon baking powder
- ½ teaspoon baking soda
- ½ teaspoon salt
- 1 ½ cup creamy peanut butter
- 1 cup packed light brown sugar
- ½ cup butter, softened
- 2 eggs
- 2 teaspoons vanilla extract
- 1 cup jelly of choice

Instructions:
- Preheat the oven to 375 degrees Fahrenheit. Grease an 8x8 inch baking dish.
- In a medium bowl, whisk together the flour, baking powder, baking soda and salt.
- In a large bowl, beat together the peanut butter, brown sugar and butter until light and fluffy. Beat in the eggs one at a time, then stir in the vanilla. Gradually beat in the dry ingredients until just incorporated.

- Spread half of the dough evenly into the prepared baking dish. Spread the jelly over the dough. Top with remaining dough, spreading it to cover the jelly.
- Bake for 25 to 30 minutes in the preheated oven, or until golden brown. Allow bars to cool before cutting into squares.

Time: 45 minutes

3. Banana Bread

Ingredients:
- 1 ½ cups all-purpose flour
- 1 teaspoon baking powder
- ½ teaspoon baking soda
- ½ teaspoon salt
- ¼ cup butter, softened
- ¾ cup packed light brown sugar
- 2 eggs
- 2 large ripe bananas, mashed
- ½ cup milk

Instructions:
- Preheat the oven to 350 degrees Fahrenheit. Grease a 9x5 inch loaf pan.
- In a medium bowl, whisk together the flour, baking powder, baking soda and salt.
- In a large bowl, cream together the butter and brown sugar until light and fluffy. Beat in the eggs one at a time, then stir in the mashed bananas and milk. Gradually beat in the dry ingredients until just incorporated.

- Pour the batter into the prepared loaf pan.
- Bake for 55 to 60 minutes in the preheated oven, or until a toothpick inserted into the center of the loaf comes out clean. Allow bread to cool in the pan for 10 minutes before turning out onto a wire rack to cool completely.

Time: 1 hour 15 minutes

4. Apple Crisp

Ingredients:
- 4 cups sliced apples
- ¾ cup packed light brown sugar
- 1 teaspoon ground cinnamon
- ¼ teaspoon ground nutmeg
- ½ cup all-purpose flour
- ¾ cup quick-cooking oats
- ½ cup butter, melted

Instructions:
- Preheat the oven to 375 degrees Fahrenheit. Grease an 8x8 inch baking dish.
- In a medium bowl, mix together the apples, brown sugar, cinnamon and nutmeg. Put the mixture into the prepared baking dish.
- In a small bowl, mix together the flour, oats and melted butter until crumbly. Sprinkle over the apple mixture.

- Bake for 40 to 45 minutes in the preheated oven, or until the top is golden brown and the apples are tender. Allow crisp to cool for 10 minutes before serving.

Time: 55 minutes

5. Strawberry Shortcake

Ingredients:

- 2 cups all-purpose flour
- 2 teaspoons baking powder
- ½ teaspoon salt
- ¼ cup vegetable oil
- ¾ cup milk
- 2 cups strawberries, sliced
- 1 cup heavy cream
- 2 tablespoons white sugar

Instructions:

- Preheat the oven to 375 degrees Fahrenheit. Grease a 9 inch round cake pan.
- In a medium bowl, whisk together the flour, baking powder and salt. In a large bowl, mix together the oil and milk until well blended. Gradually stir in the dry ingredients until just incorporated.
- Pour the batter into the prepared cake pan. Bake for 20 to 25 minutes in the preheated oven, or until a toothpick inserted into the center of the cake comes out clean. Allow cake to cool in the pan for 10 minutes before turning out onto a wire rack to cool completely.

- Place the sliced strawberries in a bowl and set aside. In a medium bowl, beat the cream and sugar until stiff peaks form.
- To assemble the shortcake, slice the cake in half horizontally. Place the bottom half of the cake on a serving plate, then top with the strawberries. Spread the whipped cream over the strawberries, then top with the remaining cake half.

Time: 45 minutes

6. Blueberry Crumble

Ingredients:
- 2 cups fresh blueberries
- ½ cup white sugar
- 2 tablespoons cornstarch
- 1 cup all-purpose flour
- ½ cup packed light brown sugar
- ¾ cup quick-cooking oats
- ¼ teaspoon ground cinnamon
- ¼ teaspoon ground nutmeg
- ½ cup butter, melted

Instructions:
- Preheat the oven to 375 degrees Fahrenheit. Grease an 8x8 inch baking dish.
- In a medium bowl, mix together the blueberries, sugar and cornstarch. Put the mixture into the prepared baking dish.
- In a small bowl, mix together the flour, brown sugar, oats, cinnamon and nutmeg. Pour in the melted butter and stir until crumbly. Sprinkle the mixture over the blueberries.

- Bake for 35 to 40 minutes in the preheated oven, or until the top is golden brown and the blueberries are tender. Allow crumble to cool for 10 minutes before serving.

Time: 50 minutes

7. Apple Oatmeal Muffins

Ingredients:

- 2 cups all-purpose flour
- 1 cup quick-cooking oats
- 1 teaspoon baking powder
- ½ teaspoon baking soda
- ½ teaspoon salt
- ¾ cup packed light brown sugar
- ½ cup butter, melted
- 2 eggs
- ¾ cup milk
- 1 cup apples, peeled and diced

Instructions:

- Preheat the oven to 375 degrees Fahrenheit. Grease a 12-cup muffin tin.
- In a medium bowl, combine the flour, oats, baking powder, baking soda, salt, and brown sugar.
- In a separate bowl, mix together the melted butter, eggs, and milk.
- Add the wet ingredients to the dry ingredients and mix until just combined.
- Fold in the diced apples.

- Divide the batter evenly among the muffin cups.
- Bake for 18-20 minutes, or until a toothpick inserted into the center of a muffin comes out clean.
- Allow the muffins to cool in the tin for 10 minutes before transferring to a wire rack to cool completely.

Time: 35 minutes

8. Banana-Yogurt Parfaits

Ingredients:
- 2 cups plain Greek yogurt
- 1 cup diced bananas
- ½ cup granola
- ¼ cup honey

Instructions:
- In a medium bowl, combine the yogurt, bananas, and honey.
- Divide the yogurt mixture among four serving glasses.
- Top each serving with ¼ cup of granola.
- Serve immediately or chill in the refrigerator until ready to serve.

Time: 10 minutes

9. Peanut Butter and Banana Oatmeal

Ingredients:
- 2 cups rolled oats
- 2 cups milk
- 2 tablespoons honey
- 2 tablespoons peanut butter

- 1 banana, sliced

Instructions:
- In a medium saucepan, bring the oats and milk to a boil.
- Reduce the heat to medium-low and simmer for 5 minutes, stirring occasionally.
- Remove the pan from the heat and stir in the honey, peanut butter, and banana slices.
- Serve warm or chill in the refrigerator until ready to serve.

Time: 15 minutes

10. Sweet Potato Muffins

Ingredients:
- 1 ½ cups all-purpose flour
- ½ cup brown sugar
- 1 teaspoon baking powder
- ½ teaspoon baking soda
- ½ teaspoon ground cinnamon
- ¼ teaspoon salt
- 1 cup mashed sweet potatoes
- ½ cup vegetable oil
- ½ cup milk

Instructions:
- Preheat oven to 375°F.
- In a large bowl, whisk together the flour, brown sugar, baking powder, baking soda, cinnamon, and salt.

- In a separate bowl, mix together the mashed sweet potatoes, oil, and milk until combined.
- Pour the wet ingredients into the dry ingredients and stir until combined.
- Divide the batter among 12 greased muffin cups.
- Bake for 20 minutes or until a toothpick inserted into the middle of a muffin comes out clean.

Time: 30 minutes

11. Apple Pie Oatmeal

Ingredients:
- 2 cups rolled oats
- 2 cups water
- ½ teaspoon ground cinnamon
- ¼ teaspoon ground nutmeg
- ¼ teaspoon ground allspice
- 2 apples, cored and diced
- ¼ cup raisins

Instructions:
- In a medium saucepan, bring the oats and water to a boil.
- Reduce the heat to medium-low and simmer for 5 minutes, stirring occasionally.
- Add the cinnamon, nutmeg, allspice, apples, and raisins to the pan and stir to combine.
- Simmer for an additional 5 minutes, stirring occasionally.
- Serve warm or chill in the refrigerator until ready to serve.

Time: 15 minutes

12. Chocolate Chip Yogurt Parfaits

Ingredients:

- 2 cups plain Greek yogurt
- ½ cup mini chocolate chips
- ½ cup granola

Instructions:

- In a medium bowl, stir together the yogurt and chocolate chips.
- Divide the yogurt mixture among four serving glasses.
- Top each serving with ¼ cup of granola.
- Serve immediately or chill in the refrigerator until ready to serve.

Time: 10 minutes

13. Apple Pie Fritters

Ingredients:

- 2 cups all-purpose flour
- 2 teaspoons baking powder
- ¼ teaspoon salt
- 1 cup milk
- 2 eggs
- 2 tablespoons melted butter
- 2 apples, cored and diced
- ½ teaspoon ground cinnamon
- ¼ teaspoon ground nutmeg
- ¼ teaspoon ground allspice

Instructions:
- In a large bowl, whisk together the flour, baking powder, and salt.
- In a separate bowl, whisk together the milk, eggs, and melted butter.
- Make a well in the center of the dry ingredients and pour in the wet ingredients. Stir until just combined.
- Add the apples, cinnamon, nutmeg, and allspice to the batter and stir until combined.
- Heat a skillet over medium heat and lightly grease with butter or oil.
- Working in batches, drop ¼ cup of batter into the skillet and cook until golden brown, about 2 minutes per side.
- Serve the fritters warm.

Time: 30 minutes

14. Peanut Butter and Jelly Oatmeal

Ingredients:
- 2 cups rolled oats
- 2 cups water
- 2 tablespoons peanut butter
- ½ cup jelly

Instructions:
- In a medium saucepan, bring the oats and water to a boil.
- Reduce the heat to medium-low and simmer for 5 minutes, stirring occasionally.

- Remove the pan from the heat and stir in the peanut butter and jelly.
- Serve warm or chill in the refrigerator until ready to serve.

Time: 15 minutes

15. Banana Oat Pancakes

Ingredients:
- 1 cup all-purpose flour
- 1 cup rolled oats
- 2 teaspoons baking powder
- ¼ teaspoon salt
- 1 cup milk
- 2 eggs
- 2 tablespoons melted butter
- 1 banana, mashed

Instructions:
- In a large bowl, whisk together the flour, oats, baking powder, and salt.
- In a separate bowl, whisk together the milk, eggs, melted butter, and mashed banana.
- Make a well in the center of the dry ingredients and pour in the wet ingredients. Stir until just combined.
- Heat a skillet over medium heat and lightly grease with butter or oil.

- Working in batches, drop ¼ cup of batter into the skillet and cook until golden brown, about 2 minutes per side.
- Serve the pancakes warm.

Time: 30 minutes

16. Yogurt Berry Popsicles

Ingredients:

- 2 cups plain Greek yogurt
- 1 cup fresh berries
- 2 tablespoons honey

Instructions:

- In a medium bowl, mix together the yogurt, berries, and honey.
- Divide the mixture among 8 popsicle molds.
- Place the mold in the freezer and freeze for at least 4 hours or until frozen.
- To release the popsicles, run the molds under warm water for a few seconds.

Time: 4 hours plus 10 minutes

17. Fruit and Nut Trail Mix

Ingredients:

- 1 cup dried cranberries
- 1 cup dried apricots
- 1 cup roasted almonds
- 1 cup roasted cashews
- ½ cup shredded coconut

Instructions:
- In a large bowl, mix together the cranberries, apricots, almonds, cashews, and coconut.
- Divide the mixture into individual servings and store in airtight containers.

Time: 10 minutes

18. Baked Apples

Ingredients:
- 4 apples, cored and sliced
- ½ cup brown sugar
- ½ cup oats
- ½ teaspoon ground cinnamon
- ¼ teaspoon ground nutmeg
- 2 tablespoons butter, melted

Instructions:
- Preheat oven to 375°F.
- In a medium bowl, mix together the brown sugar, oats, cinnamon, and nutmeg.
- Arrange the apples in a greased baking dish.
- Top the apples with the oat mixture and drizzle with melted butter.
- Bake for 20-25 minutes or until the apples are tender and the topping is golden brown.
- Serve warm.

Time: 25 minutes

19. Chocolate Chip Banana Bread

Ingredients:

- 1 ½ cups all-purpose flour
- ½ cup brown sugar
- 1 teaspoon baking powder
- ½ teaspoon baking soda
- ¼ teaspoon salt
- 2 bananas, mashed
- ½ cup vegetable oil
- ½ cup milk
- ½ cup mini chocolate chips

Instructions:

- Preheat oven to 350°F.
- In a large bowl, whisk together the flour, brown sugar, baking powder, baking soda, and salt.
- In a separate bowl, mix together the mashed bananas, oil, and milk until combined.
- Pour the wet ingredients into the center of the dry ingredients after creating a well there. Stir until just combined.
- Fold in the chocolate chips.
- Pour the batter into a greased loaf pan and bake for 35-40 minutes or until a toothpick inserted into the center of the bread comes out clean.
- Let the bread cool before slicing.

Time: 1 hour

20. Peanut Butter and Chocolate Granola Bars

Ingredients:

- 2 cups rolled oats
- ½ cup peanut butter
- ½ cup honey
- ½ cup mini chocolate chips

Instructions:

- Preheat oven to 350°F.
- In a large bowl, mix together the oats, peanut butter, honey, and chocolate chips until combined.
- Line an 8x8 inch baking dish with parchment paper and press the oat mixture into the dish.
- Bake for 15-20 minutes or until golden brown.
- Let the bars cool before cutting into bars.

Time: 35 minutes

Chapter 4: Special Dietary Needs for Seniors

Seniors with Alzheimer's disease often require special dietary needs to help maintain their health and wellbeing. As Alzheimer's disease progresses, the individual may experience changes in appetite, difficulty swallowing, and decreased ability to recognize familiar foods. In order to meet their nutritional needs, it is important to pay close attention to their dietary intake.

It is essential that seniors with Alzheimer's disease receive adequate amounts of vitamins, minerals and other essential nutrients. A balanced diet should include plenty of nutrient-dense foods such as fruits, vegetables, whole grains, lean proteins, nuts, and seeds. Eating smaller, more frequent meals throughout the day can help ensure that nutritional needs are met. To make it easier for seniors to get their daily nutrients, it is important to provide foods that are easy to eat and that are visually appealing.

It is also important to ensure that a senior with Alzheimer's disease has access to plenty of fluids throughout the day. Drinking plenty of water is important for overall health, but it is even more important for people with Alzheimer's, as dehydration can worsen confusion and other cognitive symptoms. If a senior is unable to drink enough fluids, other beverages such as juices, soups and smoothies can be used to supplement their fluid intake.

In addition to providing a balanced diet, it is important to be aware of any food allergies or sensitivities that a senior may have. For example, some seniors may have difficulty digesting lactose, so it is important to provide dairy-free alternatives. It is also important to be aware of any medications the senior is taking, as certain foods may interfere with their effectiveness.

It is also important to provide a safe and comfortable environment for seniors with Alzheimer's disease. Avoiding foods that are high in sugar, fat, and salt can help reduce the risk of overeating, while providing foods that are easy to eat can help ensure that nutritional needs are met. With the right diet and environment, seniors with Alzheimer's disease can lead healthy and fulfilling lives.

When preparing meals for a senior with Alzheimer's disease, it is important to be mindful of their personal preferences and dietary restrictions. It is also important to ensure that meals are easy to chew and swallow, and that they are not too spicy or too salty. Providing a variety of textures and flavors can help ensure that meals are interesting and enjoyable. For example, adding fresh herbs and spices to meals can help enhance the flavor and make the meal more appetizing. Additionally, offering finger foods such as cut-up fruits and vegetables can make it easier for seniors to eat and enjoy their meals.

In order to make sure that seniors with Alzheimer's disease meet their nutritional needs, it is important to offer snacks throughout the day. Providing healthy snacks such as nuts, seeds, and fruits can help ensure that seniors get enough calories and nutrients. Additionally, providing snacks that are easy to eat and enjoy can help increase food intake and maintain a healthy weight.

Finally, it is important to be mindful of any dietary restrictions that a senior with Alzheimer's disease may have. If a senior is avoiding certain foods due to allergies, sensitivities, or other health issues, it is important to provide alternatives that are both nutritious and enjoyable. With the right foods and environment, seniors with Alzheimer's disease can lead healthy and fulfilling lives.

Here are some special diet recipes to help provide different options for seniors;

Low-Sodium Recipes

1. Baked Salmon with Herbs and Lemon
Ingredients:
- 4 Salmon fillets
- 2 tablespoons of olive oil
- 2 teaspoons of fresh herbs (thyme, rosemary, oregano, etc.)
- 1 lemon
- Salt and pepper to taste

Instructions:
- Preheat the oven to 350 degrees F.
- Place the salmon fillets on a greased baking sheet.
- Drizzle the olive oil over the salmon and season with salt and pepper.
- Squeeze the juice of the lemon over the salmon and sprinkle with the herbs.
- Bake for 15-20 minutes until the salmon is cooked through.

Time: 25 minutes

2. Broccoli and Cheese Quinoa:

Ingredients:
- 1 cup of quinoa
- 2 cups of vegetable broth
- 2 cups of broccoli florets
- ¼ cup of shredded cheese

Instructions:
- In a saucepan, bring the vegetable broth to a boil.
- Add the quinoa and reduce the heat to low.
- Simmer for 15 minutes, stirring occasionally.
- Add the broccoli and simmer for another 5 minutes.
- Add the cheese and stir until melted.

Time: 25 minutes

3. Cauliflower Rice Stir Fry

Ingredients:
- 1 head of cauliflower, grated
- 1 tablespoon of olive oil
- 2 cloves of garlic, minced
- ½ cup of frozen peas
- ¼ cup of diced bell pepper
- ¼ cup of diced onion
- 2 tablespoons of soy sauce

Instructions:
- Heat the olive oil in a large skillet over medium heat.
- Add the garlic, onion, and bell pepper and sauté until softened.
- Add the cauliflower rice and stir to combine.
- Add the peas and soy sauce and stir to combine.
- Cook for 5-7 minutes, stirring occasionally, until the cauliflower is cooked through.

Time: 15 minutes

4. Egg and Spinach Omelette

Ingredients:
- 2 eggs
- 1 cup of spinach
- 1 tablespoon of olive oil
- Salt and pepper to taste

Instructions:
- Heat the olive oil in a non-stick skillet over medium heat.
- Crack the eggs into the skillet and season with salt and pepper.
- Add the spinach and scramble the eggs until cooked through.
- Flip the omelette and cook for an additional minute.
- Serve and enjoy.

Time: 10 minutes

5. Zucchini Noodles with Avocado Sauce

Ingredients:
- 2 zucchinis
- 2 avocados
- 2 cloves of garlic
- 2 tablespoons of olive oil
- ¼ cup of vegetable broth
- Salt and pepper to taste

Instructions:
- Using a spiralizer, spiralize the zucchinis into noodles.
- In a blender, combine the avocados, garlic, olive oil, and vegetable broth and blend until smooth.
- Heat a large skillet over medium heat and add the zucchini noodles.
- Sauté the noodles for 3-5 minutes until softened.
- Add the avocado sauce and stir to combine.

Time: 10 minutes

6. Baked Cod with Tomato Basil Sauce

Ingredients:

- 4 cod fillets
- 2 tablespoons of olive oil
- ½ cup of diced tomatoes
- 2 cloves of garlic, minced
- 2 tablespoons of fresh basil, chopped
- Salt and pepper to taste

Instructions:

- Preheat the oven to 375 degrees F.
- Place the cod fillets on a greased baking sheet.
- Drizzle the olive oil over the cod and season with salt and pepper.
- In a small saucepan, heat the tomatoes, garlic, and basil over medium heat until bubbling.
- Pour the sauce over the cod and bake for 15-20 minutes until the cod is cooked through.

Time: 30 minutes

7. Grilled Chicken with Mango Salsa

Ingredients:

- 4 chicken breasts
- 2 tablespoons of olive oil
- 1 mango, diced
- ¼ cup of diced red onion
- ¼ cup of diced bell pepper
- 2 tablespoons of fresh cilantro, chopped

- Juice of 1 lime
- Salt and pepper to taste

Instructions:
- Heat a grill or grill pan to medium-high heat.
- Brush the chicken breasts with olive oil and season with salt and pepper.
- Grill the chicken for 10-15 minutes until cooked through.
- In a bowl, combine the mango, red onion, bell pepper, cilantro, and lime juice.
- Serve the chicken with the mango salsa.

Time: 25 minutes

8. Herb Roasted Vegetables

Ingredients:
- 2 cups of diced vegetables (carrots, potatoes, bell peppers, etc.)
- 2 tablespoons of olive oil
- 1 tablespoon of fresh herbs (thyme, rosemary, oregano, etc.)
- Salt and pepper to taste

Instructions:
- Preheat the oven to 400 degrees F.
- Place the vegetables on a greased baking sheet.
- Drizzle the olive oil over the vegetables and season with salt and pepper.

- Sprinkle with the herbs and toss to combine.
- Roast for 20-25 minutes until the vegetables are cooked through.

Time: 30 minutes

9. Slow Cooker Turkey Chili

Ingredients:

- 1 pound of ground turkey
- 1 can of diced tomatoes
- 1 can of black beans, drained and rinsed
- 1 onion, diced
- 2 cloves of garlic, minced
- 2 tablespoons of chili powder
- 1 teaspoon of cumin
- Salt and pepper to taste

Instructions:

- Place all of the ingredients in a slow cooker and stir to combine.
- Cook on low for 6-8 hours or on high for 3-4 hours.
- Serve and enjoy.

Time: 6-8 hours

10. Stuffed Peppers

Ingredients:

- 4 bell peppers, halved and seeded
- 1 cup of cooked quinoa
- 1 cup of diced tomatoes
- ½ cup of shredded cheese

- ¼ cup of diced onion
- 2 cloves of garlic, minced
- 2 tablespoons of olive oil
- Salt and pepper to taste

Instructions:
- Preheat the oven to 350 degrees F.
- Place the bell pepper halves on a greased baking sheet.
- In a bowl, combine the quinoa, tomatoes, cheese, onion, garlic, and olive oil.
- Stuff the bell pepper halves with the quinoa mixture.
- Bake for 20-25 minutes until the peppers are tender.

Time: 30 minutes

Gluten-Free Recipes

1. Gluten-Free Buckwheat Pancakes

Ingredients:
- 1 cup buckwheat flour
- 1 teaspoon baking powder
- 1 teaspoon baking soda
- ½ teaspoon salt
- 2 tablespoons honey
- 2 tablespoons oil
- 2 eggs
- 1 cup buttermilk

- 2 tablespoons melted butter

Instructions:
- In a bowl, mix together the buckwheat flour, baking powder, baking soda and salt.
- In a separate bowl, mix together the honey, oil, eggs, buttermilk and melted butter.
- Add the wet ingredients to the dry ingredients and mix until combined.
- Heat a skillet over medium heat and spray with cooking oil.
- Pour 1/4 cup of the batter onto the skillet.
- Cook until the edges start to become golden brown. Flip and heat until the other side is golden brown.
- Serve with desired toppings.

Time: 15 minutes

2. Zucchini Fritters

Ingredients:
- 2 zucchinis, grated
- 1 teaspoon garlic powder
- 1 teaspoon onion powder
- 2 eggs, beaten
- 3 tablespoons gluten-free flour
- 2 tablespoons olive oil

Instructions:
- In a bowl, combine the grated zucchini, garlic powder, onion powder, eggs and gluten-free flour.

- Heat the olive oil in a large skillet over medium heat.
- Drop spoonfuls of the mixture into the skillet and flatten with a spatula.
- Cook for 3-4 minutes on each side, or until golden brown.
- Serve with your favorite sauce or topping.

Time: 15 minutes

3. Quinoa Salad

Ingredients:
- 1 cup quinoa, cooked
- 1 cucumber, diced
- 1 red pepper, diced,
- 1/2 cup cherry tomatoes, halved
- 1/2 cup black beans, drained and rinsed
- 1/4 cup red onion, diced
- 2 tablespoons olive oil
- 2 tablespoons white wine vinegar
- 1 tablespoon honey
- 1 teaspoon garlic powder
- 1 teaspoon cumin, salt and pepper to taste

Instructions:
- In a bowl, combine the cooked quinoa, cucumber, red pepper, cherry tomatoes, black beans and red onion.
- In a separate bowl, whisk together the olive oil, white wine vinegar, honey, garlic powder, cumin, salt and pepper.
- Pour the dressing over the salad and mix until everything is uniformly covered.

- Serve chilled or at room temperature.

Time: 20 minutes

4. Baked Salmon with Asparagus

Ingredients:
- 2 salmon fillets
- 4 asparagus spears
- 2 tablespoons olive oil
- 1 tablespoon lemon juice
- 1 teaspoon garlic powder
- 1 teaspoon dried oregano, salt and pepper to taste

Instructions:
- Preheat oven to 400°F.
- Place the salmon and asparagus on a baking sheet lined with parchment paper.
- Drizzle with olive oil and lemon juice.
- Sprinkle with garlic powder, oregano, salt and pepper.
- Bake for 20 minutes, or until the salmon is cooked through and the asparagus is tender.
- Serve with your favorite sides.

Time: 25 minutes

5. Chickpea Curry

Ingredients:
- 1 tablespoon olive oil
- 1 onion, diced
- 1 red bell pepper, diced

- 2 cloves garlic, minced
- 1 tablespoon curry powder
- 1 teaspoon ground turmeric
- 1 can chickpeas, drained and rinsed
- 2 cups vegetable broth
- 1/2 cup coconut milk
- 2 tablespoons tomato paste
- 1/4 teaspoon red pepper flakes
- Salt and pepper to taste

Instructions:
- Heat the olive oil in a large skillet over medium heat.
- Add the onion, bell pepper and garlic and simmer for 3-4 minutes, or until the veggies are soft.
- Add the curry powder and turmeric and cook for an additional minute.
- Add the chickpeas, vegetable broth, coconut milk, tomato paste and red pepper flakes.
- Bring to a boil, lower heat, and simmer for 10 minutes.
- Add salt and pepper to taste.
- Serve over cooked rice or quinoa.

Time: 25 minutes

6. Sweet Potato Soup

Ingredients:
- 2 tablespoons olive oil
- 1 onion, diced
- 2 cloves garlic, minced

- 1 teaspoon ground cumin
- 2 sweet potatoes, peeled and cubed
- 4 cups vegetable broth
- 1 can coconut milk
- 2 tablespoons maple syrup
- salt and pepper to taste

Instructions:
- Heat the olive oil in a large pot over medium heat.
- Add the onion and garlic and cook for 3-4 minutes, or until the vegetables are tender.
- Add the cumin and cook for an additional minute.
- Add the sweet potatoes, vegetable broth and coconut milk.
- Bring to a boil, reduce the heat, and simmer for 20 minutes, or until the sweet potatoes are tender.
- Use an immersion blender to blend the soup until smooth.
- Stir in the maple syrup and season with salt and pepper to taste. Serve warm.

Time: 30 minutes

7. Quinoa Bowl with Roasted Veggies

Ingredients:
- ½ cup quinoa, cooked
- ½ cup broccoli, chopped
- ½ cup cauliflower, chopped
- ½ cup carrots, sliced
- ¼ cup olive oil
- 2 tablespoons balsamic vinegar

- 1 teaspoon garlic powder
- 1 teaspoon dried oregano
- ½ teaspoon dried thyme
- Salt and pepper to taste

Instructions:
- Preheat oven to 400°F.
- In a bowl, combine the broccoli, cauliflower and carrots.
- Drizzle with the olive oil and balsamic vinegar and season with the garlic powder, oregano, thyme, salt and pepper.
- Spread the vegetables onto a baking sheet and roast for 20 minutes, or until the vegetables are tender.
- Serve over cooked quinoa.

Time: 30 minutes

8. Baked Potato Wedges

Ingredients:
- 4 potatoes, cut into wedges
- 2 tablespoons olive oil
- 1 teaspoon garlic powder
- 1 teaspoon paprika
- ½ teaspoon dried oregano
- ¼ teaspoon cayenne pepper
- salt and pepper to taste

Instructions:
- Preheat oven to 400°F.

- Place the potato wedges on a baking sheet lined with parchment paper.
- Drizzle with olive oil and season with the garlic powder, paprika, oregano, cayenne pepper, salt and pepper.
- Bake for 25 minutes, or until the potatoes are tender and golden brown.
- Serve with your favorite sauce or dip.

Time: 30 minutes

9. Lentil Stew

Ingredients:
- 1 tablespoon olive oil
- 1 onion, diced
- 2 cloves garlic, minced
- 1 teaspoon ground cumin
- 1 teaspoon ground coriander
- 1 teaspoon smoked paprika
- 2 cups vegetable broth
- 1 can diced tomatoes
- 1 cup green lentils, rinsed
- 2 carrots, diced
- 1 celery stalk, diced
- ¼ cup parsley, chopped
- Salt and pepper to taste

Instructions:
- Heat the olive oil in a large pot over medium heat.

- Add the onion, garlic, cumin, coriander and smoked paprika and cook for 3-4 minutes, or until the vegetables are tender.
- Add the vegetable broth, diced tomatoes, lentils, carrots, celery and parsley.
- Bring to a boil, reduce heat, and simmer for 25 minutes, or until the lentils are tender.
- Add salt and pepper to taste. Serve warm.

Time: 45 minutes

10. Quinoa Stuffed Peppers

Ingredients:
- 4 bell peppers, halved
- 1 tablespoon olive oil
- 1 onion, diced
- 2 cloves garlic, minced
- 1 cup quinoa, cooked
- 1 can black beans, drained and rinsed
- 1 can corn, drained
- 1 teaspoon ground cumin
- ½ teaspoon dried oregano
- ½ teaspoon smoked paprika
- ¼ cup cilantro, chopped
- ¼ cup vegan cheese
- Salt and pepper to taste

Instructions:
- Preheat oven to 400°F.

- Place the bell pepper halves on a baking sheet lined with parchment paper.
- Heat the olive oil in a large skillet over medium heat.
- Add the onion and garlic and cook for 3-4 minutes, or until the vegetables are tender.
- Add the cooked quinoa, black beans, corn, cumin, oregano and smoked paprika and cook for an additional 5 minutes, stirring occasionally.
- Remove from heat and stir in the cilantro and vegan cheese.
- Season with salt and pepper to taste. Stuff the bell pepper halves with the quinoa mixture.
- Bake for 20-25 minutes, or until the bell peppers are tender.
- Serve with your favorite sauce or topping.

Time: 45 minutes

Low-Fat Recipe

1. Grilled Salmon Salad with Lemon Vinaigrette

Ingredients:

- 2 (6-ounce) salmon fillets
- 2 tablespoons extra-virgin olive oil
- 2 tablespoons lemon juice
- 1 teaspoon honey
- 1 teaspoon Dijon mustard
- ⅛ teaspoon kosher salt
- ⅛ teaspoon freshly ground black pepper

- 2 cups baby spinach
- ½ cup sliced red onion
- 2 tablespoons chopped fresh basil

Instructions:
- Heat a large nonstick skillet over medium-high heat.
- Rub salmon fillets with olive oil and season with salt and pepper.
- Place the salmon fillets in the skillet and cook for 4 minutes on each side, or until the salmon is cooked through.
- In a small bowl, whisk together the lemon juice, honey, Dijon mustard, and salt and pepper.
- Place the spinach in a large bowl and top with the red onion and basil.
- Drizzle the lemon vinaigrette over the salad and toss to combine.
- Place the salmon on top of the salad and serve.

Time: 20 minutes

2. Baked Chicken Breasts with Spinach and Tomatoes

Ingredients:
- 2 chicken breasts
- 1 tablespoon olive oil
- ½ teaspoon garlic powder
- ¼ teaspoon onion powder
- ¼ teaspoon dried oregano
- Salt and freshly ground black pepper, to taste
- 2 cups baby spinach

- 1 cup cherry tomatoes, halved
- 2 tablespoons freshly grated Parmesan

Instructions:
- Preheat oven to 375 degrees F.
- Rub chicken breasts with olive oil and season with garlic powder, onion powder, oregano, salt and pepper.
- Place chicken breasts on a baking sheet and bake for 25 minutes, or until chicken is cooked through.
- Heat a large skillet over medium heat.
- Add spinach and tomatoes and cook until spinach is wilted and tomatoes are tender, about 5 minutes.
- Place the cooked spinach and tomatoes on a plate and top with the cooked chicken breasts.
- Sprinkle with Parmesan cheese and serve.

Time: 30 minutes

3. Egg and Spinach Scramble

Ingredients:
- 2 large eggs
- 2 tablespoons skim milk
- ⅛ teaspoon ground turmeric
- Salt and freshly ground black pepper, to taste
- 1 tablespoon olive oil
- ½ cup chopped onion
- 1 cup baby spinach
- ¼ cup shredded cheddar cheese

Instructions:
- In a medium bowl, whisk together eggs, milk, turmeric, salt and pepper.
- Heat a large nonstick skillet over medium heat.
- Add olive oil and onion and cook until onion is softened, about 3 minutes.
- Add the eggs and cook until almost set, stirring occasionally.
- Add the spinach and cook until eggs are cooked through and spinach is wilted.
- Stir in the cheddar cheese and season with salt and pepper.
- Serve immediately.

Time: 15 minutes

4. Veggie Frittata

Ingredients:
- 2 tablespoons olive oil
- ½ cup chopped onion
- ½ cup chopped bell pepper
- ½ cup chopped mushrooms
- 2 cloves garlic, minced
- 6 large eggs
- 2 tablespoons skim milk
- ¼ teaspoon dried oregano
- Salt and freshly ground black pepper, to taste
- ¼ cup shredded cheddar cheese

Instructions:
- Preheat oven to 350 degrees F.

- Heat a large nonstick skillet over medium heat.
- Add olive oil and onion, bell pepper, mushrooms and garlic and cook until vegetables are softened, about 5 minutes.
- In a medium bowl, whisk together eggs, milk, oregano, salt and pepper.
- Pour egg mixture into the skillet with the vegetables and cook until eggs are almost set, stirring occasionally.
- Sprinkle with cheddar cheese and transfer the skillet to the oven.
- Bake for 10 minutes, or until eggs are cooked through.
- Slice and serve.

Time: 20 minutes

5. Quinoa and Black Bean Stuffed Peppers

Ingredients:
- 2 large bell peppers, halved and seeded
- 2 tablespoons olive oil
- ½ cup chopped onion
- 1 clove garlic, minced
- 1 cup cooked quinoa
- ½ cup cooked black beans
- ¼ cup frozen corn
- ¼ teaspoon ground cumin
- Salt and freshly ground black pepper, to taste
- ¼ cup shredded cheddar cheese

Instructions:
- Preheat oven to 375 degrees F.

- Place bell pepper halves in a baking dish.
- Heat a large nonstick skillet over medium heat.
- Add olive oil, onion and garlic and cook until onion is softened, about 3 minutes.
- Add quinoa, black beans, corn, cumin, salt and pepper and cook until heated through, about 5 minutes.
- Spoon quinoa mixture into pepper halves and top with cheddar cheese.
- Bake for 20 minutes, or until peppers are tender.

Time: 30 minutes

6. Baked Fish with Herbed Couscous

Ingredients:
- ½ cup couscous
- 2 tablespoons olive oil
- ¼ teaspoon dried oregano
- ¼ teaspoon dried thyme
- 2 tablespoons freshly squeezed lemon juice
- 2 (4-ounce) tilapia fillets
- Salt and freshly ground black pepper, to taste
- 2 tablespoons chopped fresh parsley

Instructions:
- Preheat oven to 400 degrees F.
- Place couscous in a medium bowl and add 1 tablespoon olive oil, oregano, thyme, and lemon juice. Stir to combine and set aside.
- Heat a large nonstick skillet over medium-high heat.

- Add remaining 1 tablespoon olive oil to the skillet.
- Season tilapia fillets with salt and pepper and add to the skillet. Cook for 3 minutes per side, or until cooked through.
- Place couscous on a baking sheet and top with fish fillets.
- Bake for 8 minutes.
- Garnish with parsley.

Time: 20 minutes

7. Baked Zucchini with Parmesan

Ingredients:
- 2 medium zucchini, thinly sliced
- 2 tablespoons olive oil
- 2 tablespoons freshly grated Parmesan cheese
- 1 teaspoon garlic powder
- ¼ teaspoon dried oregano
- Salt and freshly ground black pepper, to taste

Instructions:
- Preheat oven to 375 degrees F.
- Place zucchini slices on a baking sheet and drizzle with olive oil.
- Sprinkle with Parmesan cheese, garlic powder, oregano, salt, and pepper.
- Bake for 15 minutes, or until zucchini is tender.

Time: 20 minutes

8. Baked Apples with Cinnamon

Ingredients:
- 2 large apples, cored and sliced
- 2 tablespoons melted butter
- 2 tablespoons honey
- ½ teaspoon ground cinnamon

Instructions:
- Preheat oven to 375 degrees F.
- Place apple slices in a baking dish.
- Drizzle with melted butter and honey.
- Sprinkle with cinnamon.
- Bake for 20 minutes, or until apples are tender.

Time: 25 minutes

9. Baked Sweet Potato Fries

Ingredients:
- 2 large sweet potatoes, cut into fries
- 2 tablespoons olive oil
- 2 teaspoons garlic powder
- Salt and freshly ground black pepper, to taste

Instructions:
- Preheat oven to 375 degrees F.
- Place sweet potato fries on a baking sheet and drizzle with olive oil.

- Sprinkle with garlic powder, salt, and pepper.
- Bake for 20 minutes, or until fries are crispy.

Time: 25 minutes

10. Oven Baked Chicken Breast

Ingredients:
- 2 boneless, skinless chicken breasts
- 2 tablespoons olive oil
- 2 cloves garlic, minced
- ½ teaspoon dried oregano
- Salt and freshly ground black pepper, to taste

Instructions:
- Preheat oven to 375 degrees F.
- Place chicken breasts in a baking dish and drizzle with olive oil.
- Sprinkle with garlic, oregano, salt, and pepper.
- Bake for 20 minutes, or until chicken is cooked through.

Time: 25 minutes

Sugar-Free Recipes

1. Baked Egg and Spinach Frittata

Ingredients:
- 4 eggs
- ¼ cup skim milk
- ¼ cup chopped onion

- ¼ cup diced red pepper
- 2 cups fresh baby spinach
- ½ teaspoon garlic powder
- ½ teaspoon onion powder
- ¼ teaspoon black pepper
- ¼ teaspoon dried oregano
- ¼ teaspoon salt

Instructions:
- Preheat oven to 375°F. Grease a 9-inch pie plate.
- In a large bowl, whisk together eggs and milk.
- Add onion, red pepper, spinach, garlic powder, onion powder, black pepper, oregano, and salt. Mix until combined.
- Pour egg mixture into the prepared pie plate and bake for 25-30 minutes, or until set in the center.
- Let cool for 5 minutes before serving.

Time: 35 minutes

2. Creamy Broccoli Soup

Ingredients:
- 2 tablespoons butter
- ¼ cup diced onion
- 2 cloves garlic, minced
- 2 tablespoons all-purpose flour
- 2 cups vegetable broth
- ½ teaspoon dried thyme
- ¼ teaspoon ground black pepper
- 4 cups fresh broccoli florets

- 2 cups skim milk

Instructions:
- In a large saucepan, melt butter over medium heat. Add onion and garlic and cook until softened, about 5 minutes.
- Stir in flour and cook for 1 minute. Gradually whisk in vegetable broth and bring to a simmer.
- Add thyme and pepper. Simmer for 5 minutes.
- Add broccoli and cook for 5 minutes, or until just tender.
- Reduce heat to low and slowly pour in milk. Simmer for 10 minutes, stirring occasionally.
- Transfer soup to a blender or food processor and blend until smooth.
- Return soup to the saucepan and heat through.

Time: 30 minutes

3. Lentil and Vegetable Stew

Ingredients:
- 1 tablespoon olive oil
- ½ cup diced onion
- 2 cloves garlic, minced
- ½ teaspoon dried oregano
- ¼ teaspoon ground black pepper
- 3 cups vegetable broth
- 1 cup dried lentils
- 1 cup diced carrots
- 1 cup diced celery
- 1 cup diced red bell pepper

Instructions:
- Heat oil in a large pot over medium heat.
- Add onion, garlic, oregano, and pepper and cook until softened, about 5 minutes.
- Add broth, lentils, carrots, celery, and bell pepper. Bring to a boil, then reduce heat and simmer for 20 minutes, or until lentils are tender.
- Serve hot.

Time: 25 minutes

4. Baked Salmon with Orange Glaze

Ingredients:
- 2 tablespoons butter
- 2 tablespoons orange juice
- 2 tablespoons honey
- ¼ teaspoon ground black pepper
- 4 (4-ounce) salmon fillets

Instructions:
- Preheat oven to 400°F. Grease a 9-inch baking dish with butter.
- In a small bowl, mix together orange juice, honey, and pepper.
- Place salmon fillets in the prepared baking dish. Pour orange juice mixture over the salmon.
- Bake for 10-15 minutes, or until salmon is cooked through.

Time: 25 minutes

5. Zucchini Noodles with Avocado Pesto

Ingredients:
- 2 tablespoons olive oil
- 2 cloves garlic, minced
- ½ teaspoon salt
- ¼ teaspoon ground black pepper
- 2 cups spiralized zucchini noodles
- ¼ cup packed fresh basil leaves
- ¼ cup chopped walnuts
- ¼ cup grated Parmesan cheese
- ¼ cup avocado

Instructions:
- Heat oil in a large skillet over medium heat. Add garlic, salt, and pepper and cook until fragrant, about 1 minute.
- Add zucchini noodles and cook until just tender, about 5 minutes.
- Transfer noodles to a large bowl.
- In a food processor, combine basil, walnuts, Parmesan cheese, and avocado. Process until a paste forms.
- Add pesto to the noodles and toss until combined. Serve warm.

Time: 20 minutes

6. Roasted Brussels Sprouts and Sweet Potatoes

Ingredients:
- 1 pound Brussels sprouts, halved
- 1 large sweet potato, peeled and cubed
- 2 tablespoons olive oil

- 1 teaspoon garlic powder
- ½ teaspoon onion powder
- ¼ teaspoon salt
- ¼ teaspoon ground black pepper

Instructions:
- Preheat oven to 400°F. Grease a large baking sheet with olive oil.
- In a large bowl, combine Brussels sprouts, sweet potato, olive oil, garlic powder, onion powder, salt, and pepper. Toss until vegetables are evenly coated.
- Spread vegetables on the prepared baking sheet and bake for 20-25 minutes, or until tender.
- Serve warm.

Time: 25 minutes

7. Creamy Avocado Toast

Ingredients:
- 2 slices whole-wheat bread
- 1 ripe avocado, peeled and mashed
- 1 teaspoon lemon juice
- ¼ teaspoon salt
- ¼ teaspoon ground black pepper
- 2 tablespoons fresh cilantro, chopped

Instructions:
- Toast bread until golden brown.

- In a small bowl, combine avocado, lemon juice, salt, and pepper. Mash until smooth.
- Spread mashed avocado on toast. Sprinkle with cilantro.
- Serve immediately.

Time: 10 minutes

8. Curried Chickpea Salad

Ingredients:

- 2 (15-ounce) cans chickpeas, drained and rinsed
- ¼ cup diced onion
- ¼ cup diced red bell pepper
- ¼ cup diced celery
- ¼ cup diced cucumber
- ¼ cup diced carrots
- ¼ cup plain Greek yogurt
- 2 tablespoons almond butter
- 2 tablespoons lemon juice
- 2 teaspoons curry powder
- ¼ teaspoon salt

Instructions:

- In a large bowl, combine chickpeas, onion, bell pepper, celery, cucumber, and carrots.
- In a small bowl, whisk together yogurt, almond butter, lemon juice, curry powder, and salt.
- Pour dressing over the chickpea mixture and toss until evenly coated.

- Serve chilled or at room temperature.

Time: 15 minutes

9. Roasted Veggie and Quinoa Salad

Ingredients:
- 2 tablespoons olive oil
- ½ cup diced onion
- ½ cup diced red bell pepper
- ½ cup diced zucchini
- ½ cup diced yellow squash
- ½ cup cooked quinoa
- ¼ teaspoon garlic powder
- ¼ teaspoon onion powder
- ¼ teaspoon dried oregano
- ¼ teaspoon dried thyme

Instructions:
- Preheat oven to 400°F. Grease a baking sheet with olive oil.
- In a large bowl, combine onion, bell pepper, zucchini, and squash.
- Drizzle with olive oil and add garlic powder, onion powder, oregano, and thyme. Toss until vegetables are evenly coated.
- Spread vegetables on the prepared baking sheet and bake for 15-20 minutes, or until tender.
- In a large bowl, combine roasted vegetables and quinoa. Serve warm.

Time: 25 minutes

10. Baked Apples with Pecan Topping

Ingredients:

- 4 large apples, peeled, cored, and diced
- ¼ cup rolled oats
- ¼ cup chopped pecans
- 2 tablespoons brown sugar
- 2 tablespoons butter, melted
- ¼ teaspoon ground cinnamon

Instructions:

- Preheat oven to 375°F. Grease an 8-inch baking dish.
- Place diced apples in the prepared baking dish.
- In a small bowl, combine oats, pecans, brown sugar, melted butter, and cinnamon.
- Sprinkle mixture over the apples.
- Bake for 25-30 minutes, or until apples are tender.
- Serve warm.

Time: 35 minutes

4-weeks Sample Meal Plan

Here is a 4 weeks sample meal plan that you can use to plan your meal time table in order

Week 1

Monday
Breakfast: Scrambled eggs with spinach, toast and a cup of milk
Lunch: Grilled chicken salad with a vinaigrette dressing
Dinner: Baked fish with steamed broccoli and mashed potatoes
Snack: Yogurt and fresh fruit
Dessert: Banana pudding

Tuesday
Breakfast: Oatmeal with fresh berries and a glass of orange juice
Lunch: Turkey wrap with lettuce, tomato and a side of fruit
Dinner: Baked chicken with roasted vegetables
Snack: Cheese and crackers
Dessert: Apple crisp

Wednesday
Breakfast: French toast with syrup and a glass of milk
Lunch: Grilled cheese sandwich with a side of tomato soup
Dinner: Baked salmon with roasted potatoes and asparagus
Snack: Hummus and carrot sticks

Dessert: Fruit salad

Thursday

Breakfast: Scrambled eggs with bell peppers, toast and a cup of milk
Lunch: Grilled chicken sandwich with lettuce and tomato
Dinner: Baked pork chops with steamed spinach and mashed potatoes
Snack: Trail mix
Dessert: Ice cream

Friday

Breakfast: Oatmeal with raisins and a glass of orange juice
Lunch: Grilled cheese with a side of tomato soup
Dinner: Baked fish with roasted vegetables
Snack: Yogurt and fresh fruit
Dessert: Apple crisp

Week 2

Monday

Breakfast: Scrambled eggs with spinach, toast and a cup of milk
Lunch: Turkey wrap with lettuce, tomato and a side of fruit
Dinner: Baked chicken with roasted vegetables
Snack: Cheese and crackers
Dessert: Banana pudding

Tuesday

Breakfast: French toast with syrup and a glass of milk

Lunch: Grilled chicken salad with a vinaigrette dressing
Dinner: Baked salmon with roasted potatoes and asparagus
Snack: Hummus and carrot sticks
Dessert: Fruit salad

Wednesday
Breakfast: Oatmeal with fresh berries and a glass of orange juice
Lunch: Grilled cheese sandwich with a side of tomato soup
Dinner: Baked pork chops with steamed spinach and mashed potatoes
Snack: Trail mix
Dessert: Ice cream

Thursday
Breakfast: Scrambled eggs with bell peppers, toast and a cup of milk
Lunch: Grilled chicken sandwich with lettuce and tomato
Dinner: Baked fish with roasted vegetables
Snack: Yogurt and fresh fruit
Dessert: Apple crisp

Friday
Breakfast: Oatmeal with raisins and a glass of orange juice
Lunch: Grilled cheese with a side of tomato soup
Dinner: Baked chicken with roasted vegetables
Snack: Cheese and crackers
Dessert: Banana pudding

Week 3

Monday
Breakfast: Scrambled eggs with spinach, toast and a cup of milk
Lunch: Turkey wrap with lettuce, tomato and a side of fruit
Dinner: Baked salmon with roasted potatoes and asparagus
Snack: Hummus and carrot sticks
Dessert: Fruit salad

Tuesday
Breakfast: French toast with syrup and a glass of milk
Lunch: Grilled chicken salad with a vinaigrette dressing
Dinner: Baked pork chops with steamed spinach and mashed potatoes
Snack: Trail mix
Dessert: Ice cream

Wednesday
Breakfast: Oatmeal with fresh berries and a glass of orange juice
Lunch: Grilled cheese sandwich with a side of tomato soup
Dinner: Baked fish with roasted vegetables
Snack: Yogurt and fresh fruit
Dessert: Apple crisp

Thursday
Breakfast: Scrambled eggs with bell peppers, toast and a cup of milk
Lunch: Grilled chicken sandwich with lettuce and tomato
Dinner: Baked chicken with roasted vegetables

Snack: Cheese and crackers
Dessert: Banana pudding

Friday
Breakfast: Oatmeal with raisins and a glass of orange juice
Lunch: Grilled cheese with a side of tomato soup
Dinner: Baked salmon with roasted potatoes and asparagus
Snack: Trail mix
Dessert: Ice cream

Week 4

Monday
Breakfast: Scrambled eggs with spinach, toast and a cup of milk
Lunch: Turkey wrap with lettuce, tomato and a side of fruit
Dinner: Baked pork chops with steamed spinach and mashed potatoes
Snack: Hummus and carrot sticks
Dessert: Fruit salad

Tuesday
Breakfast: French toast with syrup and a glass of milk
Lunch: Grilled chicken salad with a vinaigrette dressing
Dinner: Baked fish with roasted vegetables
Snack: Yogurt and fresh fruit
Dessert: Apple crisp

Wednesday
Breakfast: Oatmeal with fresh berries and a glass of orange juice
Lunch: Grilled cheese sandwich with a side of tomato soup
Dinner: Baked chicken with roasted vegetables
Snack: Cheese and crackers
Dessert: Banana pudding

Thursday
Breakfast: Scrambled eggs with bell peppers, toast and a cup of milk
Lunch: Grilled chicken sandwich with lettuce and tomato
Dinner: Baked salmon with roasted potatoes and asparagus
Snack: Trail mix
Dessert: Ice cream

Friday
Breakfast: Oatmeal with raisins and a glass of orange juice
Lunch: Grilled cheese with a side of tomato soup
Dinner: Baked fish with roasted vegetables
Snack: Yogurt and fresh fruit
Dessert: Apple crisp

Conclusion

Nutrition is a vital component in the health and wellbeing of seniors with Alzheimer's, and providing the right nutrition for these individuals can be a challenge for caregivers and families. Poor nutrition can lead to an increased risk of infection, weight loss, dehydration, and an overall decline in health. Proper nutrition is essential in helping seniors with Alzheimer's to maintain strength and energy while providing them with the necessary vitamins and minerals to help reduce the symptoms of the disease.

Nutrition plays an important role in helping seniors with Alzheimer's to maintain their cognitive functioning and prevent further decline. Eating a balanced diet that is rich in essential vitamins and minerals helps to support the brain and may even help to slow the progression of the disease. Antioxidants, vitamins, and omega-3 fatty acids are especially important in helping to protect against damage to the brain and reduce inflammation. Some studies have even found that dietary changes can reduce the risk of developing Alzheimer's in the first place.

Good nutrition is also important in helping seniors with Alzheimer's to maintain their strength and energy levels. A balanced diet with plenty of fruits and vegetables can provide the necessary vitamins and minerals to help support the body and prevent fatigue. Eating regular meals and snacks throughout the day can also help to maintain energy levels and prevent weight loss.

Caregivers and families of seniors with Alzheimer's should also be aware of the potential risks associated with poor nutrition. Lack of proper nutrition can lead to a weakened immune system, an increased risk of infection, and an overall decline in health. Malnutrition can also contribute to falls and other accidents.

There are many resources available for caregivers and families of seniors with Alzheimer's to help them better understand the importance of nutrition and how to provide the necessary nutrients for their loved one. The Alzheimer's Association offers a wealth of information on nutrition and provides tips for meal planning and recipes. In addition, the American Heart Association offers resources for caregivers and families on healthy eating for seniors with Alzheimer's. The National Institute on Aging also provides an online guide to nutrition for seniors with dementia.

By providing proper nutrition for seniors with Alzheimer's, caregivers and families can help to ensure that their loved one is getting the necessary nutrients to maintain their health and wellbeing. With the right nutrition, seniors with Alzheimer's can enjoy better quality of life and improved cognitive functioning.